ONE MORE BITE

HOW I OVERCAME MY FOOD DEMONS AND TOOK CONTROL OF MY LIFE

CAROLINE MATHIAS

Community with Caroline

Tulsa, OK
https://caroline.fit/

Cover and Layout Design by aspiretodesign.com

ISBN: 978-0-578-63006-9

Printed in the United Stated of America

This first book is dedicated to my husband. You allow me to be myself, 100% of the time.

Contents

INTRODUCTION

How did I get back here again?

"Here" being the place I cannot seem to escape, no matter how hard I try.

I have been writing this book for a few years now, and I keep starting over from scratch. I used to do this as a child and it drove me insane. I would write a paper and after making one mistake, would trash it and rewrite the entire thing. I am fairly certain that this nasty "all or nothing" habit has been the driving force behind my food demons that I've been battling most of my adult life. I will never stop laughing at the irony of me teaching other women how to find balance and overcome their own inner food demons. Especially tonight. I am going on my fifth year of this new lifestyle that old Caroline would have scoffed at while shoving stadium cheese fries in her face. Alas here I am, living a life of balance (finally) and finally having control of my fleeting cravings---or so I thought. It is Sunday night, and I have been "off the wagon" since Friday. I simply made my mind up on Friday that I didn't want to track anything all weekend and eat as much as I could until I was physically ill. Okay, so the last part of that was not originally in my plans, but it happened. And I sit here writing this with anger that I let myself do that again. I haven't gone off on a bender like this in a WHILE, and now I remember why. I feel like utter shit. Bloated, disappointed, confused, angry, WEAK. I hate feeling weak. It is right up there with being needy for me. I have worked my literal ass off over the past five years to feel strong, in control, self-confident, and powerful. So why do I keep letting the demons creep in and take control? Furthermore, where do they come from? I am smart enough to recognize that the reason we do anything is to evoke a certain feeling or emotion. I am also fully aware that the definition of insanity is repeating the same behavior over and over, expecting a different result, yet I was powerless to stop it for such a long time. Here is what I DO know...I'm not alone.

1

LET ME INTRODUCE YOU TO "CRAZY CAROLINE"

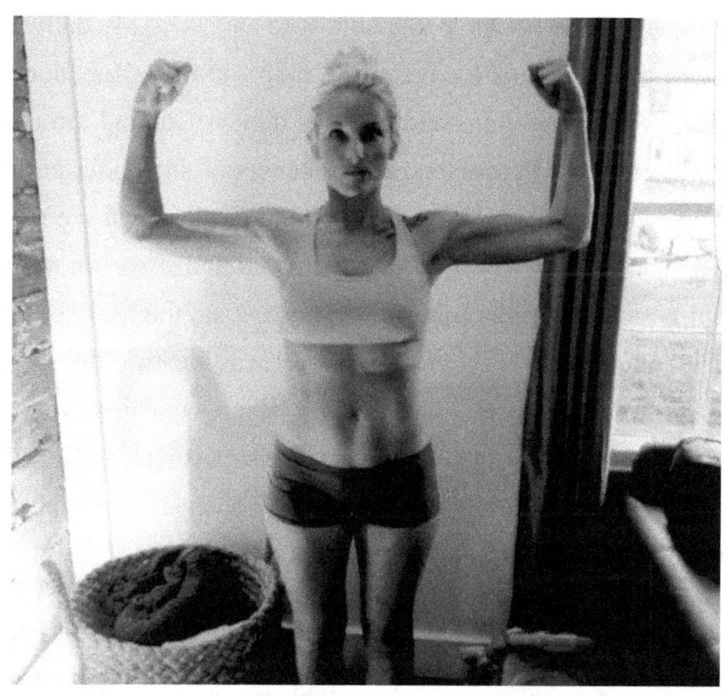

I can recall my intense love for food as early as elementary school. I studied the lunchroom menu more than I studied my classwork. I knew what day was Chili/Cinnamon roll day, and I looked forward to it like it was Christmas. I started thinking about food more than my friends and would mentally plan out my meals in advance. In middle school, there was a moment that my closest friend can still recall to this day. She said she remembers me bringing large bags of Doritos to cheer practice, and eating the entire bag before practice was over. I used to call

Doritos "cheesy chips," and they were one of my most favorite things to eat. That is until I discovered sour cream. I decided to marry the couple, and that is how my master concoction was born. (If you have never tried dipping Doritos in sour cream, I suggest you put this book down right now and try it.) To this day, I will dip salt and vinegar kettle chips in cottage cheese (add this one to your list as well). I could LIVE off of chips and dips. And I pretty much did once I moved out of my parent's house. I remember being SO excited to move in with Josh (then boyfriend, now husband) solely for the fact that I could finally go to the grocery store and buy all the shit I wanted and not have to justify it to anybody! My daily diet consisted of this: frozen pastry and oj for breakfast, chips and dips for lunch (in massive quantities) and then more chips and dips for dinner. Oh, and throughout the day, I would drink a few Dr. Peppers as well. I knew nothing about nutrition, nor did I care to. Dips were my life source, and nothing else brought me more happiness. I always say that I skated by on good genetics up until I was in my mid-twenties when the chips and dips began to reside on my ass and thighs. I spent quite a bit of time in denial about the weight gain because I was wearing the same sweatpants every day, and not leaving the house much. I began switching up my breakfast of OJ and frozen pastries for something much more sophisticated--Taco Bell. Yes, you heard me right. Taco Bell at 10 a.m. (when they opened) every morning. I would wake up, throw on my sweats, and drive to Taco Bell. I was always the only person there, so I never had to wait (bonus). I ordered two Nachos BellGrande, no beef, no beans, extra cheese, extra sour cream, extra tomatoes, and extra jalapenos. I drove home, turned on my tv, and thoroughly enjoyed my delicacy. It was bliss. I can remember these days like they were yesterday. After a few months of this, I began questioning why I was doing this on my drive each morning. It became an issue of hiding it at this point because my husband began to notice my dirty little habit--which was becoming quite expensive. In an effort to avoid questioning and utter embarrassment, I started hiding the food in the trash can. This is when I really started to feel like a winner. What in the ever-loving fuck was wrong with me? Why was I doing this? I wanted that feeling to last, that euphoric feeling that came just as I began eating, and even though I knew how short-lived it was, it still wasn't enough to make me stop. I can tell you what made me stop though--gaining 35 lbs. Once I gained so much that I physically couldn't fit in any of my clothes, and I was forced to go shopping for new ones. This was a proud moment, let me tell you. I distinctly remember standing in the dressing room trying on a size 13, that didn't fit and calling out to my mom that they must have changed all the sizes. Self-awareness was never one of my strong suits. I found myself VERY uncomfortable in my plump new bod and wanted skinny Caroline back.

Was there a stadium cheese diet?

2

OLD HABITS...LIKE EATING CHEESE FRIES...DIE HARD

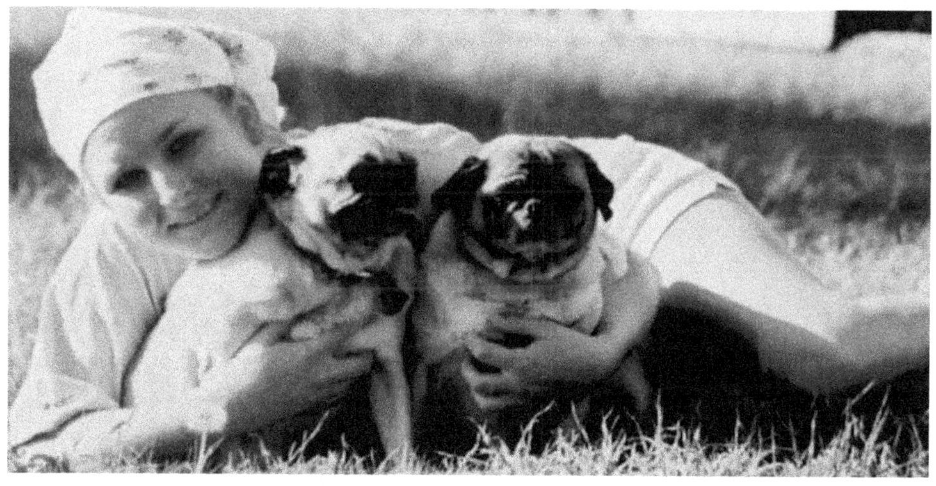

I began running and trying not to eat five bags of Doritos a day. This was the most effort that I could muster, and even then, it was excruciatingly painful. Why the FUCK would I want to eat lettuce with tuna every day? Do people really eat like this and actually enjoy it? This way of life sure as shit ain't for me, but I'll do it if the weight will come off. And the weight came off, but my food demons were still there under the surface awaiting my return. I then began a cycle of eating all that I could in one sitting, and then depriving myself for days on end. Unbeknownst to me at the time, this created a very unhealthy relationship with not just with food, but with myself. I began to self loathe, and I wasn't even aware of it at the time. **Every time I write this part I find myself rushing through it, not sure why?** Probably because I've never actually disclosed any of this all at once to anyone. I always dealt with it internally and acted fine on the outside. Moving right along, I was in this limbo of dieting on and off for a while, up until I got pregnant with my son when I was 26. I cannot explain the relief I felt when I found out I was pregnant. I thought, "this is my moment to shine." I can eat whatever the hell I want, and nobody can tell me no! I am finally fucking FREE. Fast forward nine months, and I did pregnancy proud. I gained 50 lbs and most of it was Marble Slab. I had never craved sweets in my life until I got pregnant. Then it was as if all the gallons of Blue Bell in the world were not enough. I seriously (like an idiot) thought the weight would just come off after the birth. When it didn't, and I sat on my couch attempting (unsuccessfully) to squeeze my sausage feet into my converse shoes, I burst into tears. My shoes? REALLY?! I can deal with having to wear pregnancy jeans after giving birth, that's got to be normal, but my fucking SHOES??? That was too much for me. Once I finished breastfeeding, I was ready to get the weight off for good. I would show

"YOU WILL NEVER ALWAYS BE MOTIVATED, YOU MUST LEARN TO BE DISCIPLINED."

everybody that I could do it. I started by committing to a ten day cleanse. Spoiler alert: this was the worst ten days of my life. On the bright side, I lost the last of my pregnancy weight and was starting to feel comfortable in my skin again. Alas, without having any knowledge of basic nutrition, I found myself spiraling downwards with my food demons again. Now I began experiencing some different side effects of eating whatever the hell I wanted--insane stomach issues. I had stomach aches DAILY. I kept a bottle of liquid Maalox by my bedside table and took a swig every night before bed. Instead of just changing my habits, I decided just to mask them so that I could continue eating like a complete asshole. Seems reasonable enough, right? This was Caroline logic at its finest. One specific night that I will never forget was after eating Taco Bell (again), and I was so incredibly sick to my stomach. My sister was living with us at the time, and I went upstairs to whine to her. (Josh must have been tired of hearing my shit.) I crawled up the stairs and moaned, "I am never eating like this agaaaaaaaain!" She replied, "Uh-huh..." I would do this all the time. I knew the outcome, knew that I didn't want to feel like that, but I would still follow through with the course of action. This is similar to addicts. They talk about knowing that it isn't what they want to do, but that they cannot stop. Now that I am coaching over 150 women, I have found that there is a portion of them who do not deal with issues such as this, they just need my expertise and guidance to help them reach their goals. Then I have a portion of them who are ME. If you are reading this book, then that is YOU. You will identify with every single crazed story I tell you about hiding food, binging on food, shaming myself, self-loathing, wanting so desperately to stop, but not knowing how. No matter how much you have, you will always want more. I want you to start acknowledging what you're doing, accept it, be okay with it, and move on. The dwelling and self-loathing you do is way worse than the actual act. It can be difficult to recognize on your own, and it usually takes someone who's "been in the weeds" to understand you and help you find a way out.

Our habits become our lives. If you focus on making small changes to your everyday habits, over time, those can turn into big changes in your life. You don't have to do it all at once (prob the biggest misconception ever.) When we have food issues, it is usually much deeper than food itself. Much like alcohol and drugs, we use food to cope with things that either: give us anxiety, make us uncomfortable, avoid situations, etc. The trick is that you must allow yourself to feel things and not mask them. You HAVE to begin paying attention to these triggers and figure out how to deal with them before they ruin your life. My most favorite quote that is at the bottom of all my emails is, "You will never always be motivated, you must learn to be disciplined."

3

THE CATALYST

In pretty decent shape, I got knocked up again! This time I wanted to do it differently. I knew I didn't want to bust my ass afterward getting the weight off, so I watched what I ate for the first time in my life. I only gained 25 lbs, but after giving birth, I was fully unprepared for what else was about to happen. I was staying home with my tiny humans, every woman's dream, right? Not mine. I was going crazy. I felt so out of control. I would clean all day, and by the end of the day, my house would still be a complete wreck. My husband would come home from working all day and ask me what I'd been doing and why the house was so messy. To paraphrase it for you, being a SAHM is like brushing your teeth while eating Oreos. I woke up, prepared breakfast, fed tiny humans, cleaned up breakfast, attempted to start laundry while keeping a close eye on tiny humans, so they don't waltz out into the street or shove a Lego up their butt. Shit, the laundry will just have to wait because it is time for lunch! How can tiny humans eat like truck drivers? Prepare lunch, feed tiny humans lunch, clean up lunch, try to eat something myself, get interrupted by tiny humans needing interaction, pause my lunch to play, just in time to find out they are ready for a snack. Snack time turned into mommy's wine time. I began drinking wine because it made me feel fucking great and gave me something to look forward to every day.

I want to interject here that as I am writing this, it is making me very uncomfortable because the things I was "struggling with" were not anything to be complaining about. My kids were healthy, happy, I was lucky enough to stay home with my kids, and I had an adoring husband who loved us with all his heart. I came to realize all of this shortly after I began my transformation--but this is how I felt at the time, and I feel it is important to share it in the hopes that it can help if you might be feeling helpless/lost for no apparent reason too. I realized just a few years later, after I had begun my transformation, that I was actually struggling with postpartum depression. I just didn't know it because I had been masking the confusion and pain with food and alcohol (the only way I knew how). I have also come to the realization that some women are truly meant to be SAHM's, and some aren't. I am not, and I am okay with that.

Once the drinking escalated to a bottle every night, my husband and sister stepped in (thank goodness). They gave me an ultimatum, and that is exactly what I needed. I knew I didn't want to lose my family. So I committed myself to make a lasting change--for the first time in my life.

"SUCCESS IS NOTHING MORE THAN A FEW SIMPLE DISCIPLINES PRACTICED EVERY SINGLE DAY."

You have better things on the horizon, things you may have never even let yourself dream up yet, but they are there. I promise. Commit yourself to work on yourself every day and watch what happens to your life.

4

COMPETING

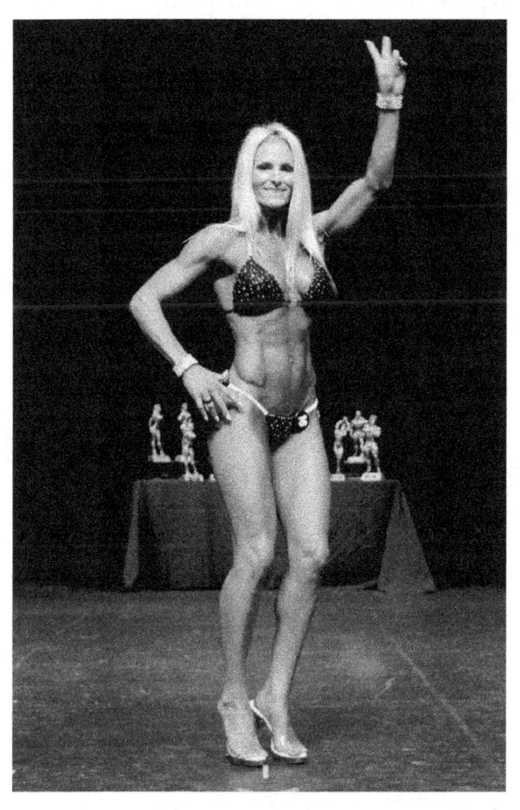

In all honesty, if I had known how much work was going to go into this transformation thing, I prob would have never started. I just knew that something had to give. When I started, I was working out almost two hours per day, seven days a week. I was eating low cal, very restrictive, and of course, I was experiencing amazing results. I had amazing coaches whom I am still close with to this day. The more weight I lost, the more self-confidence I began to experience. I had never felt like this before. Perhaps it was because I had never pushed myself or disciplined myself like this. I felt so fucking powerful every day. It became my new addiction. I went from one end of the spectrum all the way to the other. I became obsessed, but my new obsession was healthy, so what did it matter? **Sitting here writing this brings me back to this period in my life, and it's hard to recall how good I felt about myself even though I was being restrictive. ** I anxiously awaited my cheat meals, which came about every seven weeks. In the meantime, I began cheating. Nothing big, but Doritos made their appearance back in my life every night. It wasn't enough to stall my progress, so they became a staple in my diet once again (this time in moderation), and my coach never knew. You see, I never responded well to someone telling me that I couldn't have something--especially food. I was still sticking to my plan close enough, and working my ass off in the gym because I wanted more and more results. Each time I hit a goal, I set a new one. I truly believe that constantly creating new goals for yourself is the key to experiencing progress. It can be mentally demanding though, and that is why most people would rather just remain stagnant--they don't want to put in the work. I spent three years with my coaches, who came to feel like family after coaching me for my first (and last) bikini competition. I was at the point where I wanted a new challenge, and I knew this would be the biggest test of my will power--like ever. I want to preface my story of prep by saying this: I personally think that competing is a dark and twisted sport, at least for me it was. I put literally all of myself into it, expecting to win, trained the hardest I have in my life, forced my family to sacrifice, and in the end, I placed dead last and faced judgement that fucked with me terribly and took a very long time to overcome (in a nutshell). Each day began at 4 a.m., in my garage doing an hour of fasted cardio. I was eating almost 3,000 calories per day, training on my lunch break every day, with more cardio after that, working full time, and in my spare time, I was practicing posing (physically excruciating, to say the least). You put your body in positions that it is quite literally not meant to be in, so after posing, I would ache for hours. My posing was awkward AF (and I am putting that nicely). I have always been awkward...gangly. I believe I look a certain way when dancing, and then when I catch a glimpse of myself, it looks something like a dry heave set to music (name that quote). So after 12 weeks of this, I was finally ready for the stage. It would all be worth it when I won, right? Competition day arrived, and it was...odd. We all sat backstage and waited for our turn to go on. I remember feeling very out of place. And the second I stepped on stage, I knew that it was not for me. I wanted to fucking flee. I was standing there, awkward as fuck, with all these people judging my body--the body that I had worked SO hard on. I remember thinking, "who the fuck are you to tell me that I'm last place?" Once the morning show was over, I lost it. I broke down in the car and began crying uncontrollably. I was ready to go home, eat a cheeseburger and relax but I still had the night show, where all my friends and family would be watching me. I honestly didn't give a shit about anything at this point. You know that feeling when you are so over something that you lose total interest and almost laugh at the situation? That is how I felt. So I grabbed some red wine and got lit up like a Christmas tree. That was the ONLY way I was stepping on that stage again. I actually ended up placing third in the novice category, and I was okay with that. Hell, at least they recognized me for something. I thought the hard part was over. I was ready to get back to LIFE. Little did I know that I would have to "reverse diet," which means slowly adding calories back in (slowly being the keyword). SIX WEEKS OF THIS HORSESHIT. But I did it, only because I lived in constant fear of what would happen to my physique if I didn't abide by the rules. The mental agony that I experienced over the next few months was brutal. I would wake up, hop on the scale, and if it were up ½ lb, I would have an anxiety attack over it. I was obsessing about food all over again. It had all come full circle, and I wanted off the ride.

What I would tell someone wanting to compete:

Ask yourself why you want to compete. What do you think you will get out of it? If it's winning, why is winning so important to you, and what do you think it will bring you? (Spoiler alert: it won't bring you happiness, neither will washboard abs.) Ask yourself what you REALLY want, my bet is that it isn't meal prepping 20 lbs of chicken per week, avoiding social outings with your friends because you can't take a sip of alcohol, and doing 2+ hours of cardio EVERY DAY(yes, 2+ hours every damn day).

5

THE COMMUNITY

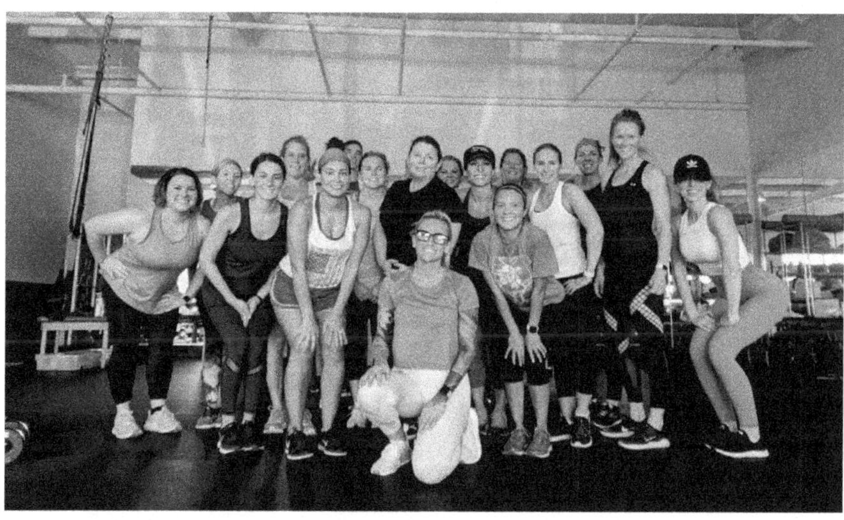

When would I just be able to live a normal life and enjoy the foods I loved? Was that even possible? What would happen if I put on a little weight and lost the body I worked so hard for? These are some of the questions I began asking myself after I decided to "go on my own" with my diet. I was excited, yet terrified at the same time. I wasn't sure if I could trust myself to make good decisions without having to check in with my coach every day. It has been almost two years since I made that decision, and it has been the best decision I made because I've learned so much about myself and what works for me in the process. I've also created a business from it called "Community with Caroline." I was recently able to quit my full-time job to coach women on how to achieve the body they want by NOT restricting their favorite foods, and the irony is still not lost on me. I want for other women what I want for myself--to eat all the yummy things while still making progress and not miss out on their life in the process. I started making changes to the Community that I was personally struggling with. If I went on a bender on the weekend, I would do a video on Monday about the importance of forgiving yourself instead of beating yourself up over it. The response from the women was overwhelming, and I learned that sharing my story with them was helping them more than having a coach order them around from a pedestal of perfection. I continue to share my struggles with them to this day, so we are all going through it together, learning from each other, and offering support when one of us is battling. I hate being cliche, but the Community has changed my life just as much as it has changed anyone else's. I desperately needed support from women who truly understood what I was going through.

Rules of the Community:

1. Nothing is off-limits.
2. If you fall off plan, get right back on. NO GUILTING OR SHAMING YOURSELF.
3. No binging
4. If you happen to binge, it's OKAY! Again, try to recognize WHY you are binging and allow yourself to sit with those emotions, and don't be afraid to ask for help!
5. No labeling foods! No bad or good, it is all just food!
6. If you want something and find yourself beginning to fixate on it, HAVE IT! Make sure it is a small portion, sit down, eat it SLOWLY (no rushing through it), acknowledge what you are doing, and ENJOY IT. Then get right back on track.

6

MINDSET

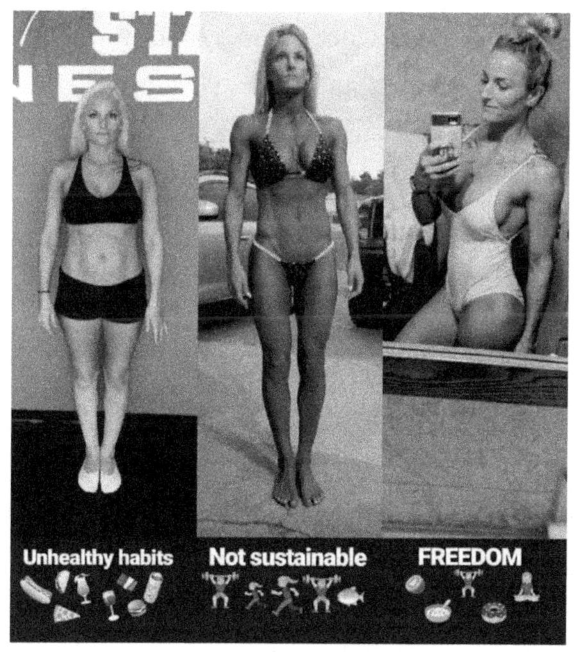

Sunday, August 4th, 2019: fresh off a 3-day bender where nothing was off-limits, I ate when I wasn't hungry, and now I sit here writing to you all feeling like a failure all over again. It is easy for me to preach to others about the importance of never allowing these negative thoughts to creep in, but the fact is they still do from time to time. I want to find that drive again. I want to channel it again.

Monday, August 5th, 2019: It is absolutely INSANE what one good day on plan can make you feel like. I did amazing today, and my mood has done a complete 360. I feel elevated (if that makes sense). I feel lighter. My stomach isn't pissed off at me. I went to the gym and got a workout in (which always helps). The main thing is that I made my mind up last night to hold myself accountable from here on out. Does that mean being perfect? FUCK NO. I will never again go into a Monday with the thought of anything being off limits, and that goes for cocktails, donuts, chips, etc. I find that when I have that restrictive outlook in my brain that it causes me to focus even harder on those things and the fact that I "can't have them." On the flip side, when I fully allow myself to do whatever I please, I suddenly don't need those things anymore. I encourage you to begin thinking like this if you struggle with food demons--it has been the driving force in the Community since I implemented the "no restrictions" policy. It is basically reverse psychology, and it FUCKING WORKS.

Mindset plays such a huge role in implementing new habits and actually sticking with them when times get tough. Anyone can start a diet and toss in the towel two weeks in when shit gets rough (which is the exact point that most people quit). I get it. You've been starving yourself and force-feeding yourself chicken and rice for 14 days (which feels like 14 years when dieting), and you haven't lost a pound. In fact, you've GAINED weight. So what is the point? In your mind, there isn't one. Why would you choose to be miserable if you aren't even going to lose weight in the process? This is precisely my reasoning behind the "no restrictions" rule. By simply allowing you to do as you please, you suddenly feel as if you aren't on a diet at all, and you aren't. You are given a meal plan with FREEDOM in it for the first time in your life. It is now up to you to execute. It's amazing how long people can stick to things that aren't miserable AF. This gives the process the time it needs for results to take place. Then the magic happens. The weight comes off, the body begins to build muscle, clothes fit differently, and you are eating donuts in the process. It is truly magical when I read client's text messages of shock and excitement when they finally realize it doesn't have to be a horrible, shitty process. Get your mind right, and you've literally won half the battle.

My personal tips for keeping your mindset tight AF:

Write shit down. Make a vision board of what you want out of life, even if it's not all physical! Keep a journal of how you are feeling day to day, especially when you fall off track. Identify the exact emotion you were feeling when it happened. Try to recognize these emotions before they start to unravel

in the future and sit with them instead of using food to comfort or suppress them. When you actually allow yourself to FEEL emotions, you grow. It can be unpleasant in the moment, but that unpleasant feeling is actual growth happening--so acknowledge it and embrace that shit. I grew the most I have in my entire life the 12 weeks I was on prep. I am thankful that I went through it for that reason alone. I am able to coach differently now because I know that everybody has the potential to be disciplined. Again, if a junk food junkie like me can do this, then I truly believe that you can too!

7

WHY YOU NEED A "WHY"

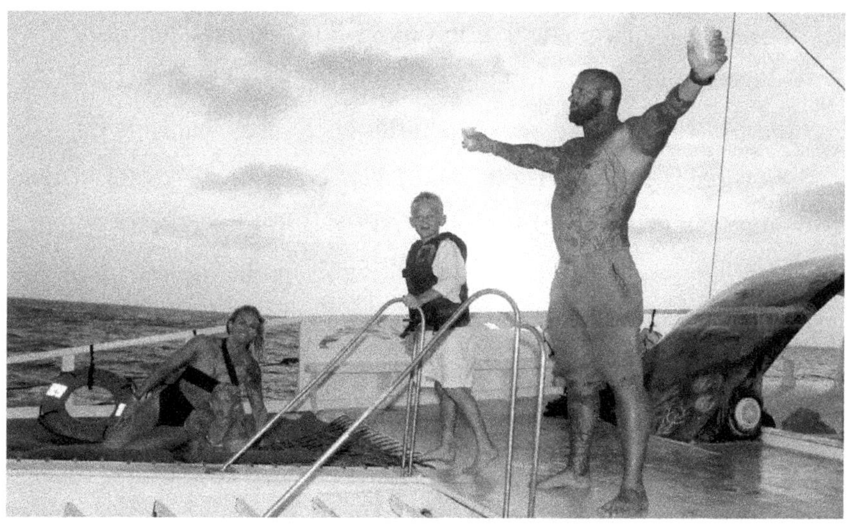

When I began my transformation, I remember being asked to find a picture of my "vision" for myself. I scoured Pinterest and looked at so many tight asses I couldn't see straight. I finally found a picture of a ballerina styled photo of this hot ass chick with the most perfect legs and butt I'd ever seen. That is what I wanted. I took a photo of my cellulite packed thighs and sent it to my coach, along with the vision pic. I told her, "I wanted my legs to no longer resemble a shattered glass window." Fast forward five years, and I can tell you that all the work I have put in has paid off tenfold, and I am happy with my body. Most days. I still have those days where I nitpick myself, but I have spent so much time rewiring my brain that I no longer sit in those moments and let them fester. It's just not a useful way to spend my time. So I realize I left a lot of gray area there with those five years, and I'm about to tell you why. In the beginning, my "why" was I wanted to look better naked, or so I thought. I ended up getting asked over and over what the real reason was behind starting my fitness journey. After about 10 min of responding with physical answers, I was forced to answer the toughest question I'd ever been asked... "Why did you feel the need to change your body? What was wrong with the way you looked?" I held back because in my opinion, talking about feelings is right up there with eating broccoli; it's physically painful and makes me quite nauseated. I answered, "I didn't like who I was on the inside." I was then asked, "WHY?" Jesus buddy, wouldn't it be easier just to give you a vile of my blood? Lord knows that would be less painful. I held back tears and uttered, "I was weak, I didn't make good decisions, and I was consciously aware of that--and I wanted to break the cycle." THERE! YA HAPPY?! But the questions kept coming until I was sobbing and talking about my drinking problem, how it had begun to affect my marriage, all of my other relationships, and most importantly, it was putting my family in jeopardy. My self-confidence was non-existent, and I desperately wanted to feel better about myself--because I KNEW that I had way more to offer in life than this. THIS was my "why." I knew that committing to myself would finally set forth the changes in my life I had so desperately wanted. Finally, I realized why I was doing all of this, and now I had a newfound sense of how I wanted to run the Community. I put more effort into each meal plan, adding shit loads of variety, and encouraging the women to begin speaking/thinking to themselves the way I wanted to speak to myself. I wanted them to forgive themselves if they fell off track. I wanted them to start speaking aloud things they loved about themselves daily. I told them to take the pressure off, that they were in a place where they were safe, and could work on loving themselves while also working on improving their bodies and minds. I vowed that I would do all of this with them, and right then and there, stop speaking negative words to myself, and I haven't since that day. This is probably the thing that I am most proud of above everything else. The feedback I have received since has been moving, to say the least. I feel like I am actually making an impact on these women's lives, and I knew I had it in me all along. Discipline has ultimately brought out my greatest strength, and I think it's because everyone who knew the old Caroline knew of her undying love for nacho cheese, and if I can do this, then dammit ANYONE CAN!

Tips for how to figure out your "why"

1. Be 100% honest with yourself.

2. Each time you answer a "why" question, ask yourself another. Like peeling back an onion layer by layer.

Ex: Why do I want to lose 20 lbs? To be thinner.

Why do I want to feel thinner? To feel comfortable in a bathing suit.

Why do I want to feel more comfortable in that bathing suit? To feel sexy, I no longer feel sexy.

Why do I want to feel sexy? So that my husband will find me more attractive.

Why do you feel like he doesn't find you attractive now? I don't know, he doesn't look at me the same, and we don't have sex much anymore. I am worried he may leave me.

Why do you think he would leave you? We have been arguing, and I want to connect with him like we did when we first met.

What has been causing the arguments? Well, I don't feel comfortable in my skin anymore, so I don't initiate sex, and that is very important to him (most all men).

DO YOU SEE WHERE THIS ALL WENT? IT IS ALWAYS DEEPER THAN THE PHYSICAL ASPECT...

Once you know your "why" you will be able to tap into a deeper feeling of your reasoning for doing this, thus helping you make better decisions because your literal life is at stake, not just having a nice ass. My entire life has changed for the better, all of my relationships have changed for the better, and my marriage is strong AF, I could go on. But that can all change if I don't continue to put the work in. This is why keeping your mindset strong is of the utmost importance!

8

CHEERLEADERS ARE OVERRATED

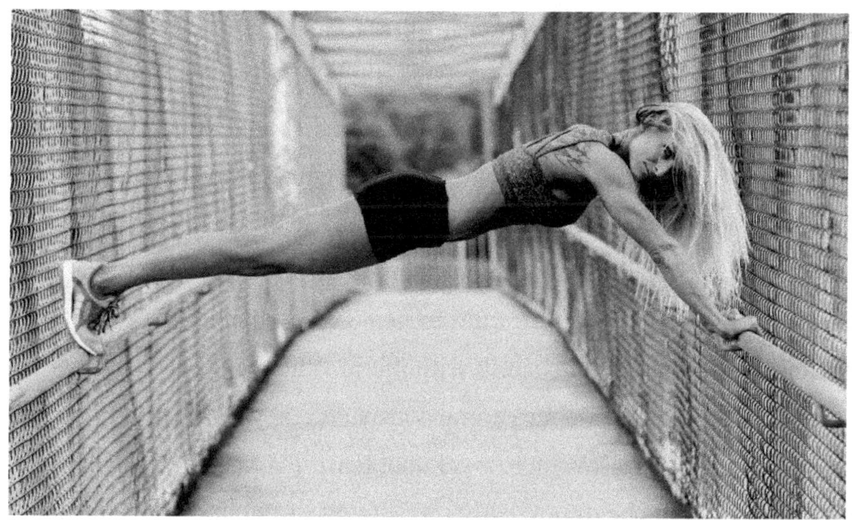

I decided to write about this because it was something that happened during the beginning of my transformation that I was not prepared for. I expected to have all of this support from my friends and family, and that is not what happened. I had friends ask me how I was going to go all summer without drinking. My parents would poke fun at me when we would have dinner at their house asking, "You can't eat CHICKEN WINGS?" I would go to birthday parties and bring a prepped meal and get the most bizarre looks. I couldn't figure out why it was such a big deal that I was trying to turn my life around and be healthier. But when you challenge yourself and do something out of character that requires work and discipline, it scares others at first. They are forced to look inside themselves and all of a sudden they aren't good enough because they aren't doing it. I felt very alone during the first year of my transformation. I rarely left the house because I was terrified of being at a restaurant and not being able to control myself when food came to the table. I wasn't really incorporating a new lifestyle, I was making progress physically but becoming more and more anti-social, which was a pretty tough feat for me already. As much as I love being alone, I couldn't live like this forever, I wanted to be able to enjoy dinners and bbq's with my friends and family. I wanted desperately to learn how others did. How did they have a few bites and stop when they were satisfied? I wanted that. I was never able to stop if I liked something; I wanted more and more and would eat until I made myself sick. Alas, I powered on, sometimes taking it one meal at a time. The more progress I saw, the more it fueled me. You see, once you begin to make REAL progress, then everyone begins to notice. You start receiving compliments and questions on how you are doing it. You think to yourself, "there really is no trick, I just do the same thing every day, and to everyone's surprise, it is actually pretty boring." People want to hear of some amazing trick that you've learned, and they want you to share it with them. When you tell them that you have simply been working hard and remaining consistent, they lose interest. Do you know why? Because people don't want to work that hard. THAT is the truth. I didn't want to work that hard in the beginning either. I just sort of put myself into autopilot, and to be quite honest am shocked as hell that I sit here writing this five years later. It all comes back around to habits. I've simply created daily habits and repeated them over and over for so long that it is my new normal. I don't particularly care to feel like complete dogshit, either. The digestive issues that I used to battle every night are non-existent unless I take it too far, and then I am reminded of how horrible it is all over again. At the end of the day, the only one who can change your life is you. Don't expect everyone to hop on your journey and be supportive, because that may not happen. While it can be discouraging, KEEP GOING. Remember that once you get some time under your belt and make some serious progress, those same people will be coming to YOU asking for help. I guarantee it.

9

KEEPING BUSY TO STAY ON TRACK

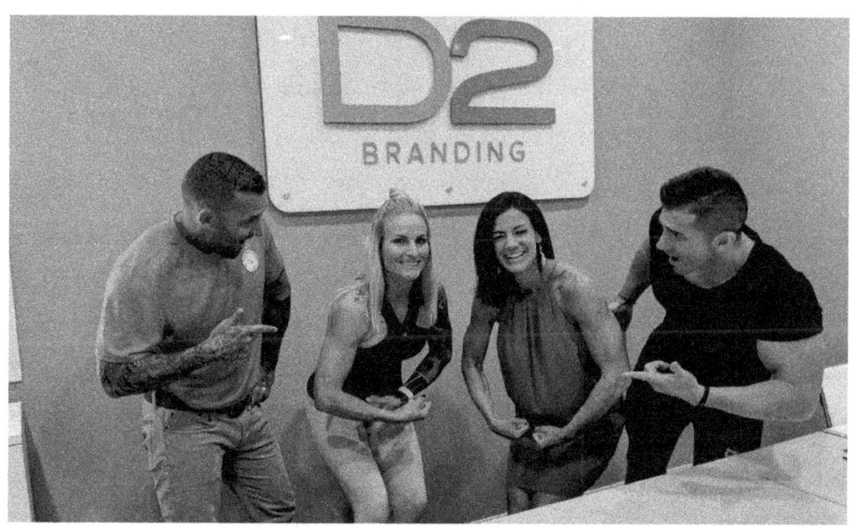

This is one of the best-kept secrets to staying on plan while also changing your life for the better--two birds. Productivity. I know it's another boring subject, but let me tell you how it has helped me turn my life around while reaching my goals, quite literally. At the beginning of my transformation, I would find myself at the house, bored and beginning to obsess about food. The more I fixated on a certain item, I eventually had to have it. I struggled with this for a while until I began to sidetrack my thoughts when I felt them becoming obsessive. I would literally go do a load of laundry, and once I had it folded, the craving was gone. I wasn't even really hungry. I was bored. If I wanted to stay on plan and my family had ordered pizza for dinner, I would go take a hot shower while they ate. Once the smell of fresh pizza is gone, and it is just warm pizza, it is amazingly less appealing. Taking small breaks from these thoughts is incredibly helpful, AND you will get so many other things done that you normally would put off. Writing this chapter is keeping me preoccupied and focused on something bigger than myself, like you reading it and learning ways to help yourself. When I say that my entire life changed once I became disciplined, this is how I did it. I became productive. I started doing things with my time that would have been spent shoveling chips in my face, not that it wasn't enjoyable. I did things that were hard and that weren't as satisfying, but the rewards were much greater. Let me tell you a story about my hopes and dreams five years ago. I wanted a farm with lots of animals. I wanted a big white house that resembled a barn. I wanted lots of land for my kids to run and play. I wanted to be my own boss. I DESPISED working for other people from the moment I had my first job at Pepper's Grill. I always had issues with authority. I wanted to do my work on my terms and make enough money to buy what I wanted when I wanted. I could not have been further from any of these things back then. I was a SAHM, struggling to "keep up with my friends," feeling like I wasn't contributing to anything, falling into the pits of depression fueled by alcohol, overweight, and trapped in a body that I felt wasn't mine. I can honestly remember dreaming of all those things and wondering if I could ever have them. When I began my journey, I knew the physical parts of me would change, but I never dreamed that every single thing that I had been wishing for would actually happen. It is all a result of discipline, hard work, consistency, and patience. If you can take anything away from this book--write those things down. I know it isn't flashy, but it is how I truly changed my life. I am sitting in my barn style white house as I write this to you, on 60 acres sprawling with cows, goats, pigs, a camel (yes, a fucking camel), donkeys, bulls, a tortoise, dogs, etc. I am working from home while my kids play upstairs. I am my own boss, doing something that I truly love for the first time in my life. My relationship with my husband has changed for the better, and we are closer now than we ever have been. I feel accomplished and grateful every single day that this is my life. I dreamt about it for so long that some mornings I wake up and literally pinch myself.

MY TIPS FOR STAYING BUSY TO KEEP YOURSELF ON TRACK TO ACHIEVE YOUR BEST LIFE:

1. When you find yourself focusing on food, distract yourself by doing something productive like laundry, dishes, a task you've been putting off, writing your thoughts down on paper, taking a hot shower, etc.

2. Make a vision board. It doesn't have to be a big production; it can literally be a small sheet of paper that you write down a few things that you want to accomplish in life. Keep it handy and look at it when you are feeling weak.

3. Remember that the time it takes you to eat something is ALWAYS 5 min or less. I use this trick to this day to keep me on plan. The time you spend planning a cheat will be more satisfying and long-lived than the act of actually sitting down and eating it. THINK ABOUT THAT.

4. Plan ahead! If you mentally plan what you are going to eat, you are more likely to stick with that and stay on track. Physically preparing meals ahead of time will also help keep you on track! If it is in your fridge, you've likely put time and effort into it already and will be more likely to have that instead of some random junk in your pantry!

5. This doesn't really have anything to do with being productive, but it's a good tip that just popped in my head. Remember that there is no perfect way to do this. Find a way that works best for YOU and do that. Whether it is eating two large ass meals per day or 5-6 small ones, it doesn't matter as long as you are hitting your daily macros! If that means saving up all your fats and carbs during the day so that you can splurge and have ice cream after dinner--DO IT! My best piece of advice is and always will be to do what works for you, your lifestyle, your job, because the easier you make it on yourself, the more likely you will be to stick with it, and at the end of the day, it is the consistency that brings results. Think about that.

10

SMALL BITES

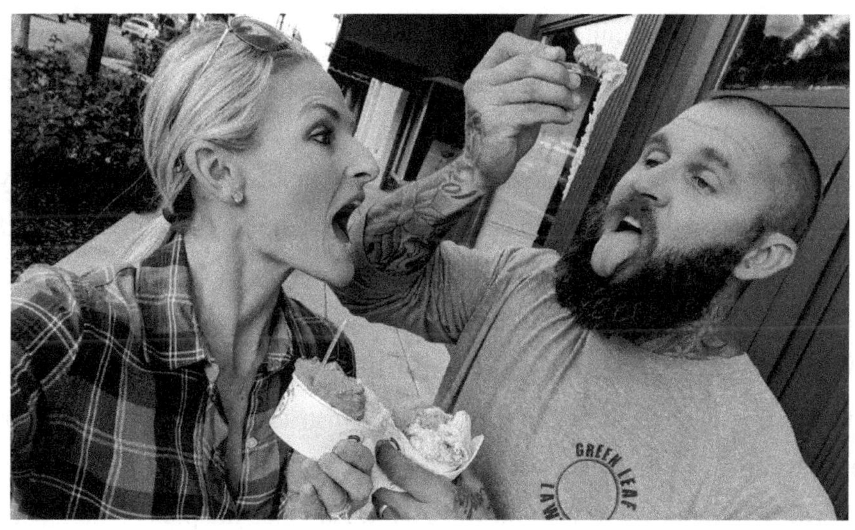

You are getting ALL of my secrets here! Small bites are something that was always discouraged by my other trainers. I never abided by most rules and made up my own as I went (as long as I was on plan 80-85% of the time it really didn't seem to matter). When I say "didn't matter," I mean that unless you are competing for a competition, there really is no sense in attempting to be perfect 100% of the time. Do you know why? Because perfection doesn't fucking exist. And the more pressure you place on yourself to be perfect, the more times you fail. Because if one thing falls out of place (which it will), then you give up completely, feeling like an utter failure. What is the point? You've fucked up already. You can't commit and just make it one damn day--so you justify a binge and vow to start again tomorrow. This cycle continues until you go absolutely insane and give up altogether, leaving you right back at square one. Sound familiar? I did this for YEARS. I never knew there was this amazing middle ground. The key is you have to accept yourself where you are at currently. You can't obsess about how far you have to go. You can't stand in the mirror, pinching every roll or patch of cellulite on your body and expect for things to magically fall into place when it's gone. Because it might not ever go away.

Now back to the small bites. Small bites have been a complete lifesaver for me and the women of the Community. The theory is that if you are craving something, have it! That's it! Now, this doesn't mean every single craving, just the ones where you are worn down and really in need of a pick me up. I just had one. My most favorite chips, salt and vinegar kettle chips. I had a small handful and put them away. It is extremely satisfying, and you still stay on track! When you discipline yourself with your serving size, the act of eating becomes infinitely more enjoyable. Because there is no guilt. You are still on your way to your vision while eating chips. WHO KNEW? This can work at parties, events, BBQ's, any place where you are going to be tempted with an array of different foods. I instruct my ladies to have a protein shake on the way so that they get their protein in first. Then at the party, make a SMALL plate and put whatever you want on it. But once the plate is done, be done. Don't eat past the point of being full--there is never a reason and you will NEVER feel good about yourself after doing it. I truly believe in having the freedom to do what you want, and the result of that will be you making better decisions.

11

FLIPPING THE SCRIPT... AND EATING DONUTS

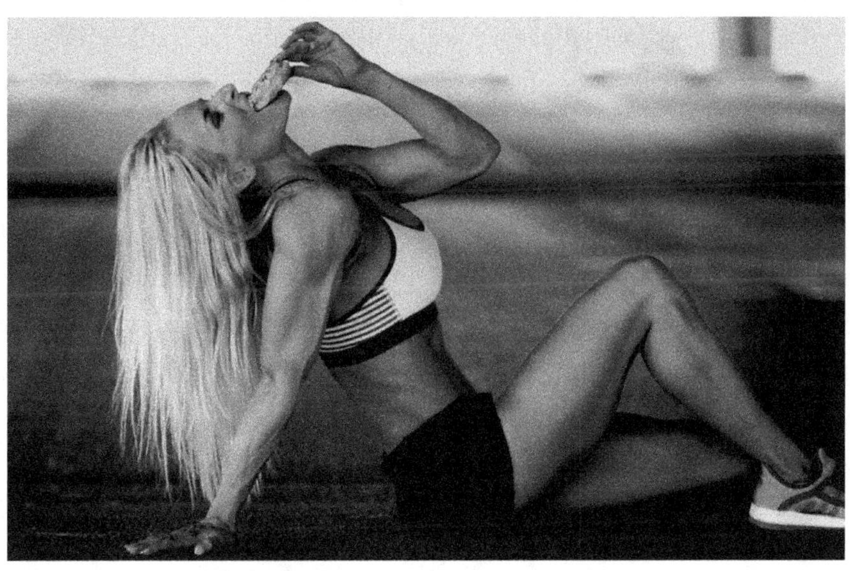

Do you know how many times I've been told not to eat things like donuts by different coaches? Too many to count, that's how many. Something had to change. It has since been my mission in life to be the first coach to spearhead this movement. First of all: a life without donuts is not worth living. Second of all: who the fuck is actually gonna swear off something as delicious as donuts for the rest of their lives? Not me, I can assure you. I can remember the second I was told not to have a certain item when dieting, and it was like I instantly had to have it. All I did was think about that one item. It became my golden unicorn, irresistible. Here is what happened: I avoided it for as long as I could until I hit a speed bump (stress, bad day at work, anxious, tired, or just plain didn't give a fuck). Guess what my thought process was on this day? "I'm going to have donuts because I DESERVE them." It was like I was punishing myself all those days restricting them and then a giant middle finger to my coach when I cheated with them. When I cheated, I went hard. I didn't just have one. I had six. This left me in terrible pain, full of shame and guilt, anxiety over admitting to my coach what I'd done, blah blah blah. I love donuts, I don't want to feel ashamed when I eat them, and nor should YOU. This is why ALL of my clients are allowed donuts and anything else they want for that matter. Once I gave them the green light to this new way of living, they truly began to thrive, and I felt damn good about my methods. They were building a better relationship with food as well as with themselves. They immediately stopped thinking of certain foods as "bad" or "good." All foods were free game. They could have them whenever they damn well pleased. And THAT was the kicker, they suddenly didn't need them that much, because I took the golden unicorn aspect away. They weren't this taboo thing anymore, so incredibly amazing that they had the potential to pack 80 lbs on you for eating just one. It's a fucking donut. Another thing I noticed not only with myself but with all my girls was that when we DID choose to have something of our liking, we didn't eat like we were going to the electric chair. We enjoyed a small portion and got right back on track because we still wanted to reach our goals!

I leave you with this final word: you are stronger than food. Food is just food. Stop giving it this power over you. The most important lesson I've learned over the past five years is that I spent so much of my life being a prisoner to food and not truly living. I let it control situations, my mood, and because of this, it ruled my entire life. Life is too short to be spent obsessing about food. If you want it, have it; but you must TRULY enjoy it and be okay with it. That is the step that most people are missing, and it is the key to overcoming food demons.

MY TIPS FOR ALLOWING YOURSELF TO ENJOY THE FOODS YOU TRULY LOVE

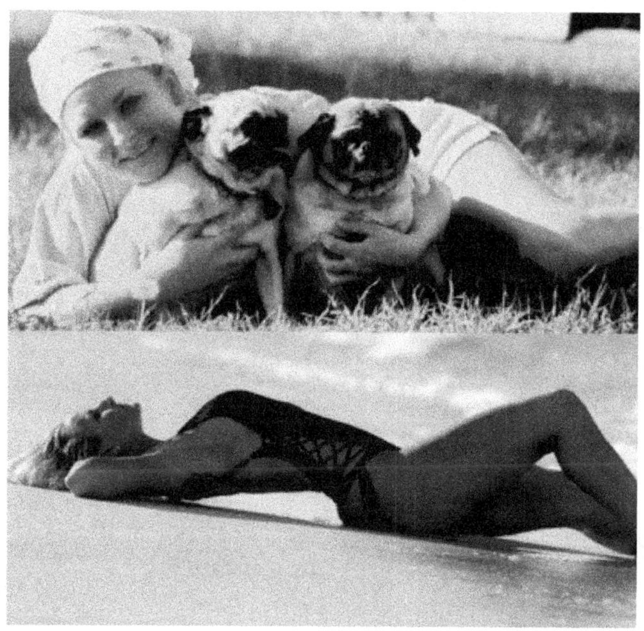

1. Implement a "no restrictions" policy with your meal plan.
2. Write down a list of your non-negotiable items (items you are absolutely not willing to live without) and make a way to add those into your everyday plan so that you are constantly looking forward to your meals. Looking forward to your meal plan is the best way to make a lasting change!
3. When you feel fearful of eating something for any reason, sit down and write down what you are feeling and why. Dissect the feeling and figure out why you feel anxious eating that item. Figuring these things out is SO important for your progress mentally as well as physically.

4. Wake up, look in the mirror, and state three things that you love about yourself. (Does not have to be a physical aspect.)

5. When you choose to have one of your fave items, sit down with a reasonably sized portion, eat it SLOWLY, and acknowledge what you are doing (eating a food that you love, that brings you true joy--and THIS IS OKAY)!

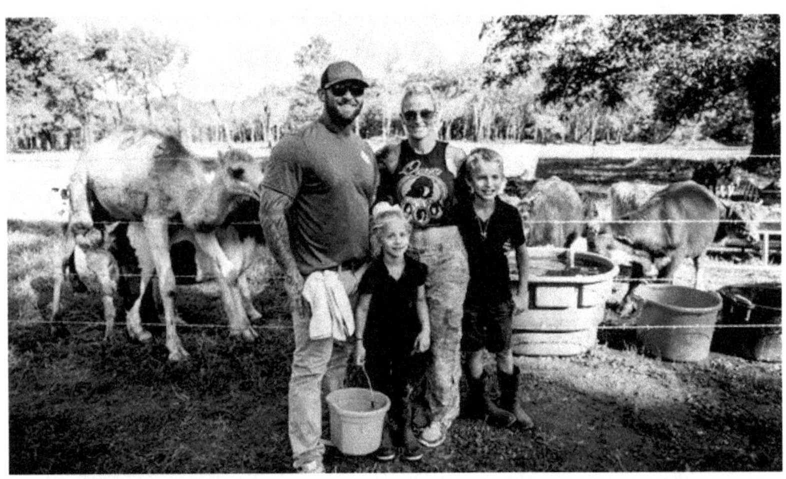

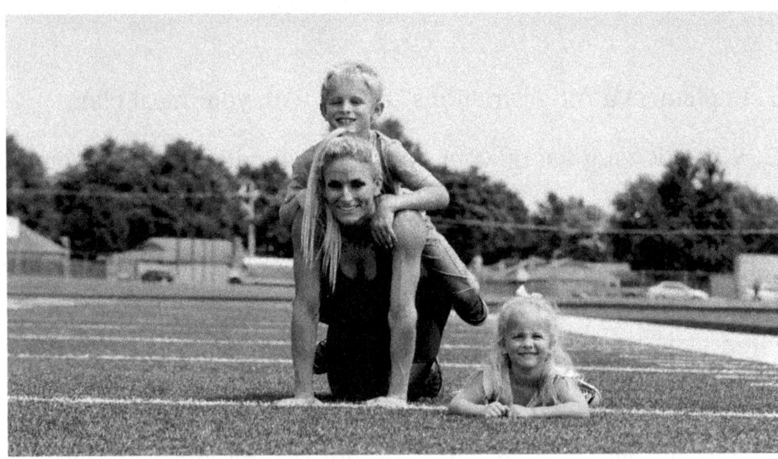

To join our Community visit: https://caroline.fit
Facebook: https://www.facebook.com/caroline.mathias.5
Email: hello@caroline.fit
Instagram: @carolinecmathias

THE MOMENT YOU'VE ALL BEEN WAITING FOR...

RECIPES!

One of the most common questions I get asked (aside from "what do you eat every day?") is, "Will I be able to eat with my family at night?" The answer to that is YES. I ate alone for three years until I finally realized how dumb it was, and consequently, what a bad example it was setting for my kids to see their mom eating separately each night. So in the Community, we fit ANYTHING in, and that includes dinner time with your family! Without further ado, here are some of my family's all-time favorite recipes!

Here are some of my staples that remain on my weekly rotation!

BREAKY:

Collagen peptides | Egg whites | Overnight Oats

Cereal | Frozen waffles

SNACKS/LUNCHES:

Turkey bacon w/hummus | PB&J

Low-fat cottage cheese w/chips (cheddar & sour cream or salt & vinegar kettle chips)

Low-fat, low-sugar greek yogurt (my fave brands are YQ, Chobani, Oikos triple zero, & fat-free Fage)

Kind brand granola | Egg whites & cereal

Nugobars | Protein shakes

Tuna Pasta Salad (see recipe on page 63)

Deli turkey wraps w/hummus, cheese, or honey mustard

DINNERS:

Casseroles (I've included a few of my favorites!)

Taco Bueno copycat burritos (tortilla, sour cream, cheese, and refried beans)

Bell & Evans frozen coconut chicken with buffalo sauce (Whole Foods)

Protein shake

Tacos

Crockpot Chicken

INGREDIENTS

2-3 lbs Boneless Skinless Chicken Breast

2 packets of Ranch seasoning mix

Seasoned salt

1 cup Salsa verde (any green salsa will do)

Fat Free Fage yogurt

DIRECTIONS

1. Place all ingredients except yogurt in slow cooker and cook on high for 2-3 hours.
2. Remove chicken and shred with Kitchenaid mixer.
3. Add in 1/2 cup-1 cup of fat free Greek yogurt to make creamy!

*This will be your most used recipe, because it is so versatile and can be used in many of the recipes in this book!

CHANGE YOUR LIFE *Chili*

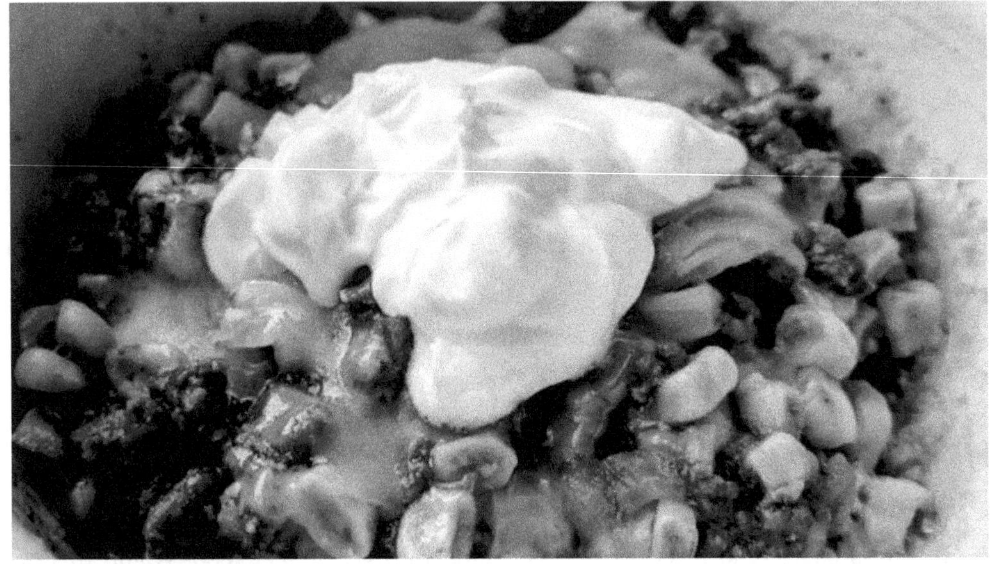

INGREDIENTS

1 lb ground beef, bison, or turkey

1-15 ounce can white or yellow corn

1-11 ounce can white corn

1 can mild Rotel

2 cans petite diced tomatoes

Tomato paste (as needed)

1 yellow onion

Garlic, Seasoned salt, Salt

1 tbsp Unsweetened dark chocolate (This is the secret ingredient!)

DIRECTIONS

1. Season beef with seasoned salt (lots) Cook until brown.
2. Cook diced onion with a few tbsp of fresh or minced garlic until softened (almost translucent). I add a little bit of oil if needed, and salt!
3. Add beef and onions to crockpot, along with all other ingredients.
4. Cook on low for 4-6 hours or on high for 2-3.

Recipe inspired by: Fawna Anderson

ADDITIONAL TOPPINGS (OPTIONAL)

Cheese of choice (I like Rico's)

Light sour cream

Low-fat cottage cheese

Jalapenos

Scallions

Fritos (or any chips you like)

"THE CAROLINE WAY"

Rico's nacho cheese

Light sour cream

Cornbread

Jalapenos (nacho slices)

Salt and vinegar kettle chips

MACROS FOR A 10OZ SERVING WITHOUT TOPPINGS: 20C/10F/15P

Taco Mac

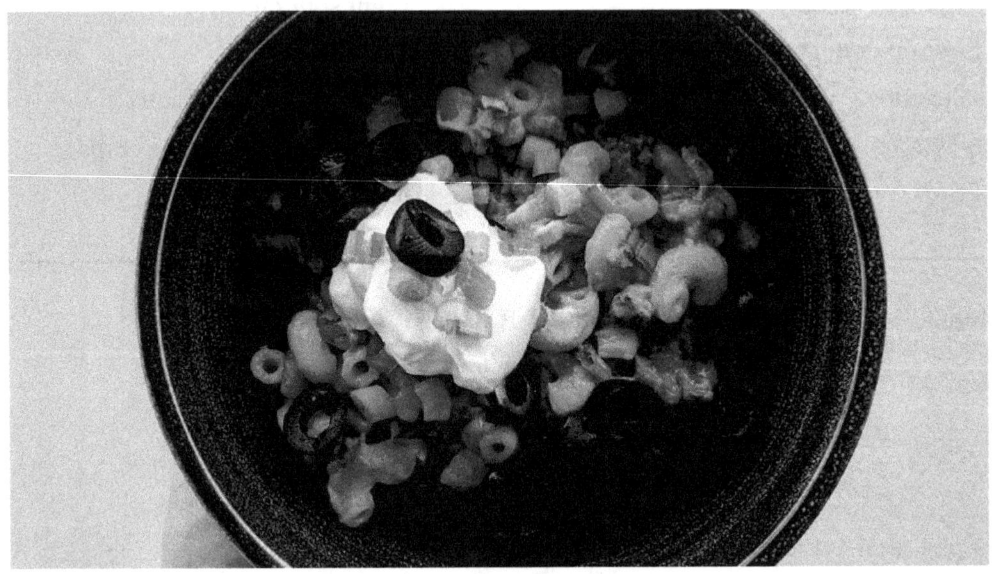

INGREDIENTS

10 oz macaroni noodles

1 lb 90% lean ground beef (you could even use ground turkey to lower the fat content!)

1/4 cup diced onion

1 tbsp minced garlic

1 cup salsa

1 packet Cheesy taco seasoning

8 oz 1/3 fat cream cheese

1/2 cup shredded Monterey Jack, 1/2 cup sharp cheddar (combine them after shredding) **you could also buy the pre-shredded cheese but that shit grosses me out to be honest)

1.5 cups Mexicorn

DIRECTIONS

1. Preheat oven to 375. Spray a 9x13 baking dish with cooking spray.
2. Cook your macaroni and set aside.
3. Cook your meat and then drain the fat. Add onions and garlic and cook until the onions are translucent. Add the taco seasoning and salsa and mix!
4. Add ground beef mixture to the noodles and place on low heat. Add the cream cheese and 1/2 cup of the cheese mixture. Mix until fully melted and pour into baking dish.
5. Add the remaining 1/2 cup of cheese to the top and bake for 15 min.
6. Optional toppings: black olives, cilantro, light sour cream, lettuce, scallions.

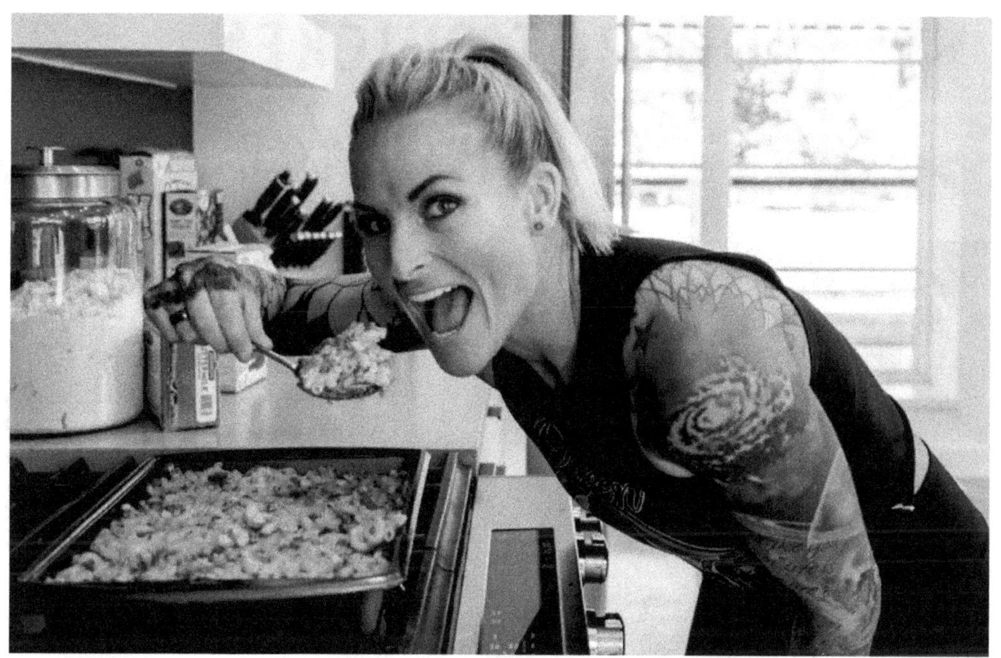

This is one of those "stand over the baking pan and eat until you can't see straight" recipes (obviously--see above). It is RIDICULOUSLY good! But it's also a great family dinner that everyone will love, and you can enjoy as well!

Recipe adapted from: http://thediaryofarealhousewife.com

MACROS FOR 4 OZ SERVING WITH NO TOPPINGS: 20C/7/10P

MACROS FOR 8 OZ SERVING WITH NO TOPPINGS: 40C/14F/20P

***YOU COULD SAVE UP SOME OF YOUR CARBS DURING THE DAYTIME, AND HAVE YOURSELF A LARGE 8 OZ SERVING OF THIS AND MEET YOUR MACROS PERFECTLY!**

CROCKPOT CHICKEN
Air Fried Tostadas

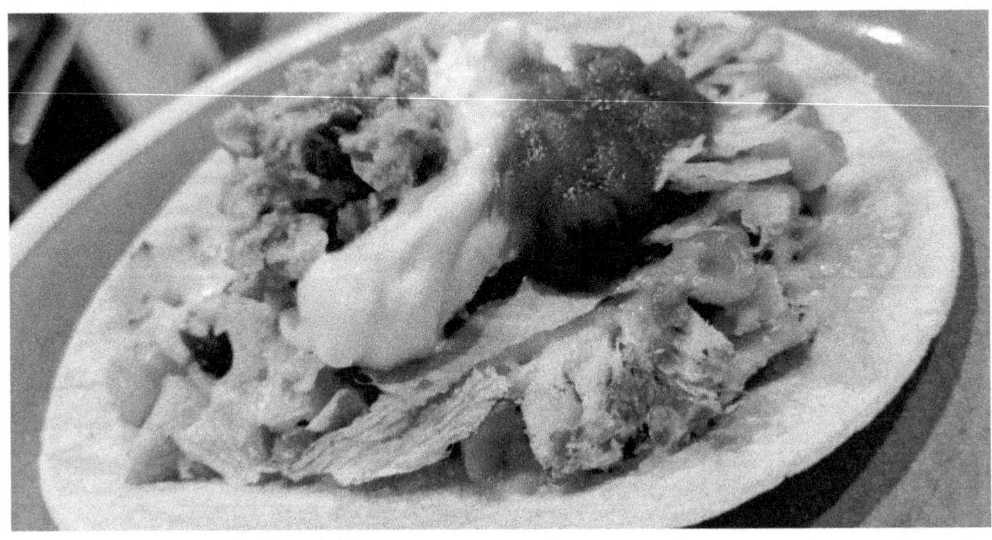

This is a super quick, delicious, family friendly meal that everyone can enjoy! It can also be whipped up as a quick and easy lunch if you are in a hurry!

If you prep the crockpot chicken ahead all you have to do is assemble the tostadas and air fry at 375 for 5 min! Make sure you add the chicken to the tostadas BEFORE placing in the fryer, and then add all other ingredients when they are done!

Pictured: 3 oz Caroline's Crockpot Chicken, 2 small corn tortillas, 2 tbsp Trader Joe's corn salsa, lettuce, salsa, 1 tbsp light sour cream, 1/3 avocado, cilantro

SMOKIN' HOT *Tilapia*

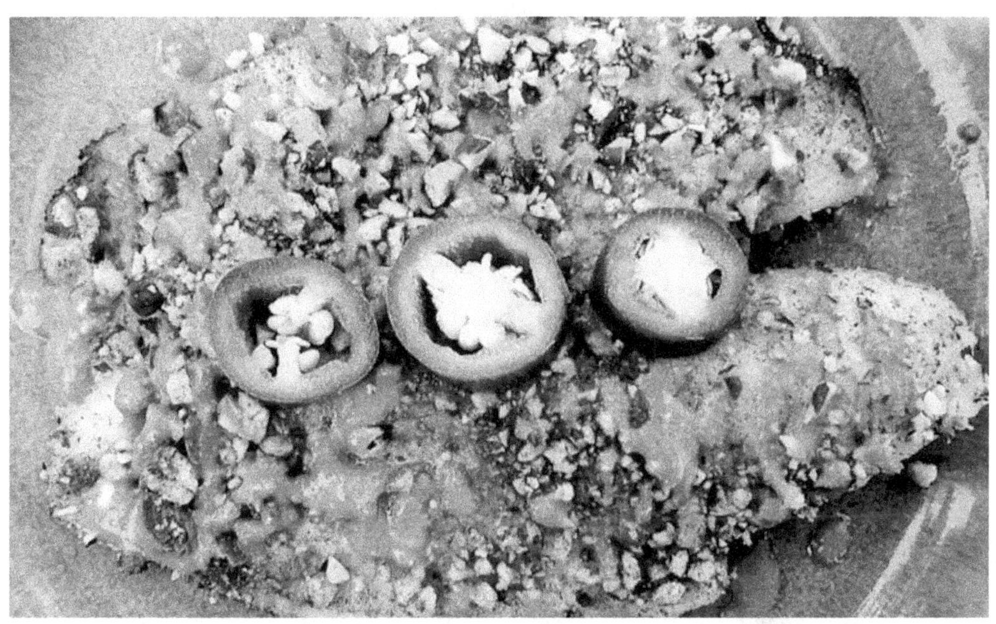

INGREDIENTS

Tilapia or Cod

Smoked Paprika

Salt N Vinegar Almonds

Fresh Jalapenos

Sriracha

Fat free Fage yogurt

Lime juice

DIRECTIONS

1. Coat fish with crushed almonds/paprika mixture.
2. Bake at 400 for 12 minutes if using Tilapia. Broil 3-4 inches from heat for 10-12 minutes if using Cod.
3. Mix sriracha, Fage and lime juice, then drizzle over fish.
4. Top with fresh jalapenos and lime juice!

DA BOMB
Frito Chili Pie

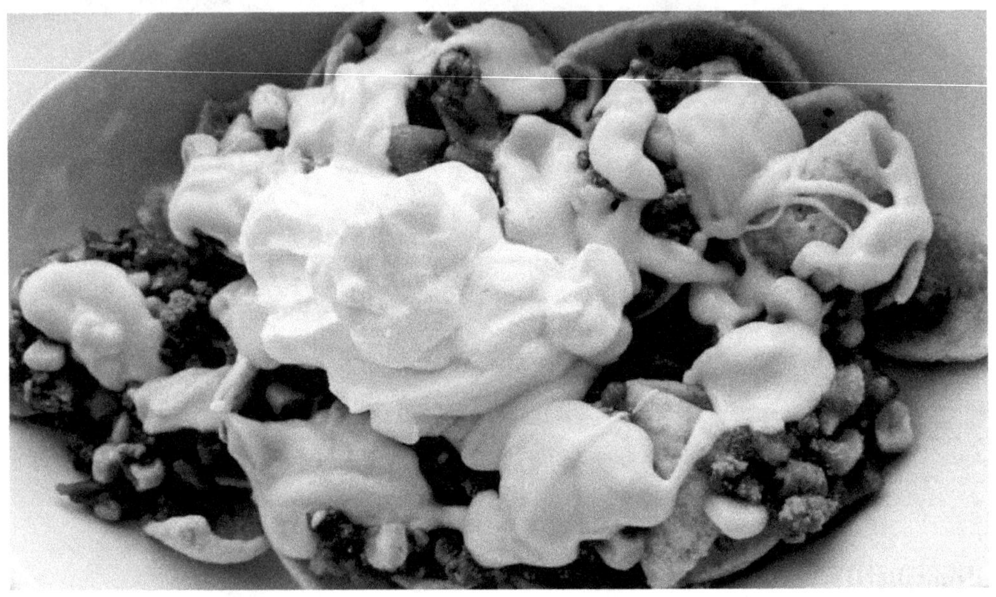

INGREDIENTS

1/2 cup Change Your Life Chili (recipe on page 44)

10 Fritos Scoops

2 tbsp light sour cream

1/8 cup Ricos nacho cheese

This is yet another recipe that if you made Change Your Life Chili for meal prep or dinner, then you can toss this bad boy together in less than 5 minutes! As far as it being a well-balanced meal in terms of the ratio of protein, carbs, and fats--it def meets the mark! The Chili is low in fat so that gives you more room to splurge on the chips, cheese, and sour cream!

CILANTRO LIME *Rice*

INGREDIENTS

2 cups sushi rice (measured dry)

2 tsp salt

1 tbsp olive oil

4 tbsp finely chopped cilantro

3 tbsp fresh lime juice

3 tbsp fresh lemon juice

2 tbsp orange juice

DIRECTIONS

1. In a medium saucepan over high heat, bring water to a boil.
2. Add rice and salt. Stir to coat rice. Return to a boil.
3. Once it is a full rolling boil, reduce to simmer and cover for 20 minutes.
4. Remove from heat and leave covered for 5 minutes.
5. Add the salt, oil, cilantro, and juices. Stir to combine. Serve and enjoy!

Recipe adapted from: www.theslowroasteditalian.com

AIR FRIED *Chicken*

INGREDIENTS

Boneless skinless chicken breasts or tenders

Sea salt and vinegar almonds (Sprouts)

Egg whites

DIRECTIONS

1. Slice breasts up so that they have more mixture on each piece!
2. Dip chicken strips into egg whites, then into pureed almonds, place into air fryer.
3. Fry at 350 for 18 minutes.

LINDSAY'S
Hamburger in a Bowl

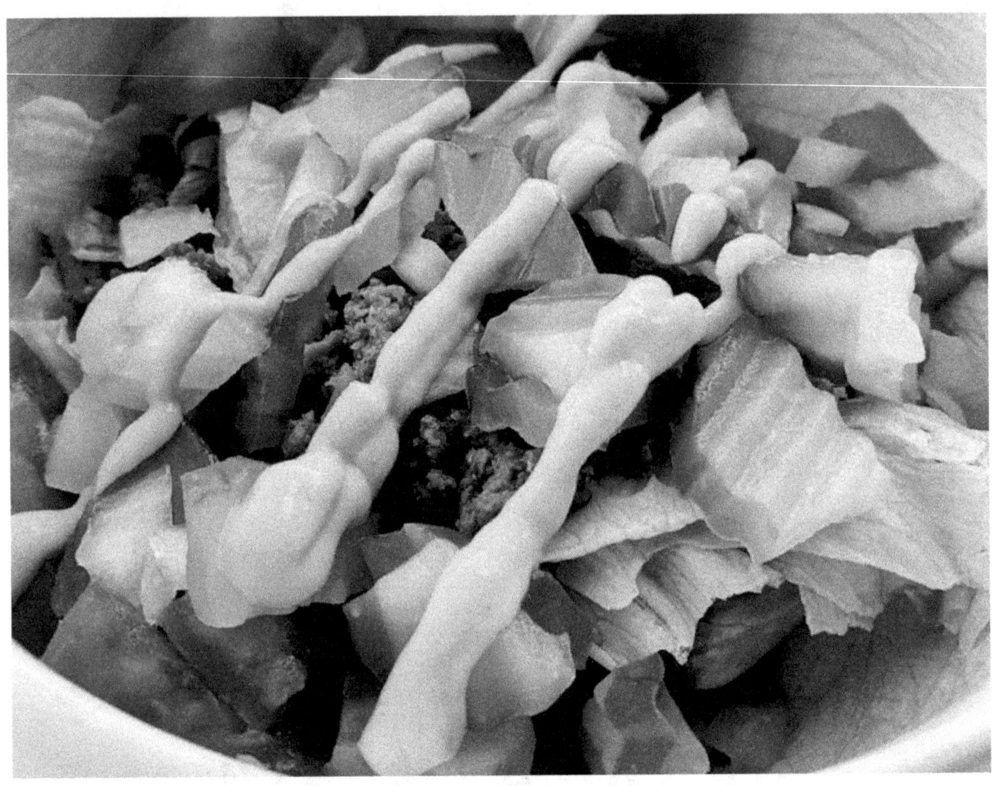

INGREDIENTS

3-4 oz of lean hamburger meat (90/10)

1 cup of lettuce

4-6 cherry tomatoes

diced onions

2 pickles, chopped

Top with mustard

DIRECTIONS

1. Combine all ingredients in a bowl and devour!

This is a recipe that one of my clients created, and it is one of the best ones that all of my clients make to this day!

Recipe by: Lindsay Burk

THE MOST MOIST GLUTEN FREE Turkey Meatloaf

INGREDIENTS

8 ounces mushrooms, trimmed and very finely chopped

1 medium onion, peeled and finely chopped

2 garlic cloves, peeled and minced

1 tablespoon oil, 1 teaspoon kosher salt, 1/2 teaspoon ground black pepper, 1 tablespoon Worcestershire sauce, 7 tablespoons low sugar ketchup(divided)

1 cup (60 grams) brown rice cereal, blended

1/3 cup (80 ml) unsweetened almond milk

2 large eggs, lightly beaten (may use egg whites too)

1 1/4 pound extra lean ground turkey (98% lean)

Recipe from:
www.inspiredtaste.net

DIRECTIONS

Prepare meatloaf

Heat oven to 400 degrees F. Lightly oil a rimmed baking sheet (or 9-inch by 13-inch baking pan) lined with aluminum foil. Heat oil in a large skillet over medium-low heat. Add the onion and cook, stirring occasionally, until softened; about 5 minutes. Add the garlic and cook until fragrant, about 1 minute. Stir in the mushrooms, a 1/2-teaspoon of salt, and a 1/4-teaspoon of pepper. Cook until the mushrooms give off their liquid and it boils away; about 10 minutes. Transfer the onions and mushrooms to a large bowl, and then stir in the Worcestershire sauce and 3 tablespoons of the ketchup. Set aside to cool for 5 minutes. Meanwhile, combine the cereal crumbs and milk in a small bowl. Stir the cereal crumb mixture and the eggs into the mushrooms and onions. Using a fork or your hands, gently mix in the turkey, a 1/2-teaspoon of salt, and a 1/4 teaspoon of pepper. The mixture will be very wet. Form the meatloaf into a 9-inch by 5-inch oval in the middle of the prepared baking sheet. Spread the remaining 4 tablespoons of ketchup on top.

Bake meatloaf

Bake the meatloaf until an instant read thermometer inserted into the thickest part of the meatloaf registers 170 degrees F, about 50 minutes. Let stand 5 minutes before slicing.

MESSY *Tacos*

INGREDIENTS

1 lb ground turkey or extra lean ground beef

1 packet cheesy taco seasoning mix

2/3 cup water

La Tiara taco shells

Lettuce

Fat free Fage yogurt

Frank's Red Hot

Salsa

DIRECTIONS

1. Brown meat until cooked, and then add the taco seasoning packet with 2/3 cup water.
2. Once blended together, top your tacos with the meat, lettuce, and salsa.
3. In a separate bowl, mix a small amount of Fage with the Red Hot and some salsa. Top your tacos! YUM!

SWEET & SPICY *BBQ Chicken*

INGREDIENTS

Grilled chicken (You could also use Crockpot Chicken but it tastes better using grilled.)

Red onion

Sugar free BBQ sauce (1 ounce)

Ranch dressing (1 tbsp)

Rice (any kind)

Jalapenos (optional)

DIRECTIONS

1. Grill your chicken using lemon pepper seasoning, seasoned salt, and low sodium soy sauce
2. Combine cooked chicken with rice, BBQ sauce, red onion, ranch dressing, and jalapenos!

BUFFALO CHICKEN *Salad*

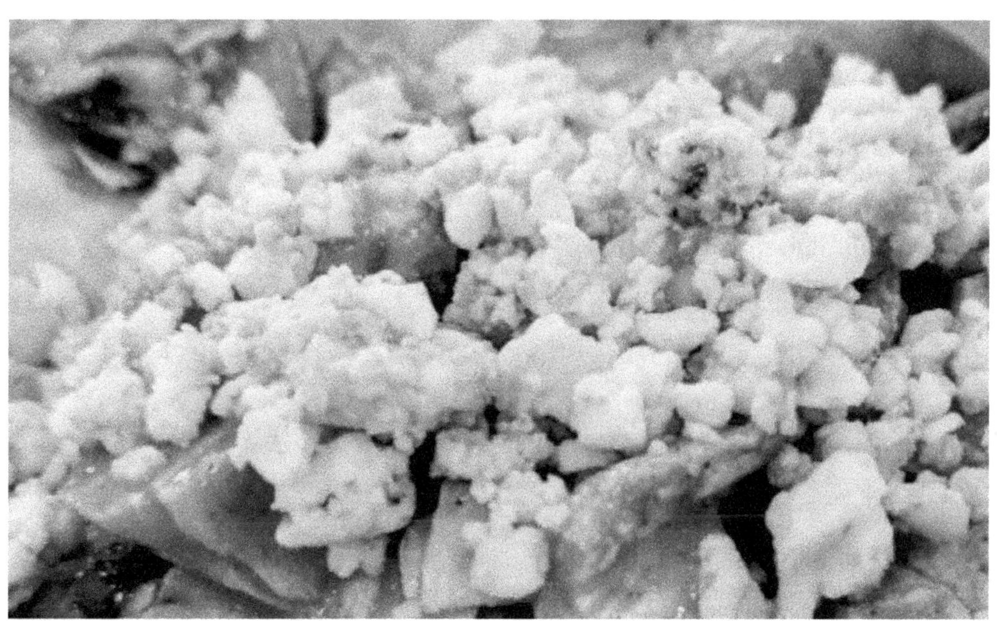

INGREDIENTS

Grilled chicken (You may also use the Crockpot Chicken for this!)

1 oz of blue cheese crumbles

Romaine

Wing time sauce

1-2 tbsp of Blue Cheese dressing

DIRECTIONS

1. Combine all ingredients and enjoy!

You may also sub ranch dressing for the blue cheese and regular cheddar cheese for the blue cheese!

This is my go-to when I am struggling at dinner time!

BBQ *Street Tacos*

INGREDIENTS

Your serving size of Crockpot Chicken (recipe on page 43)

Slaw - 1/2 c fat free greek yogurt, lime juice, lemon juice, salt & pepper, paprika, shredded cabbage, scallions, cilantro

BBQ sauce

2 small corn or flour tortillas

DIRECTIONS

1. Top each tortilla with some chicken, a spoonful of slaw, and a drizzle of BBQ sauce!

EGG WHITE *Muffins*

INGREDIENTS

1 carton of egg whites

Optional add-ins: Baby spinach, chopped onion, chopped red pepper, chopped jalapeno, chopped turkey bacon, chopped ham, chopped mushrooms, sriracha sauce

Recipe from: hemandhers.blogspot.com

DIRECTIONS

1. Preheat oven to 350 degrees.
2. Spray muffin pan, and add chopped ingredients to each cup. Add about 1/3 cup liquid egg whites per cup.
3. Bake for 30 minutes. Immediately remove and let cool on a rack.
4. Once cool, place 2 in ziploc bag with no air to keep them all week in the fridge.
5. To reheat, remove from bag and heat in microwave for 1 minute and enjoy!

AVOCADO SHRIMP
Ceviche Tostadas

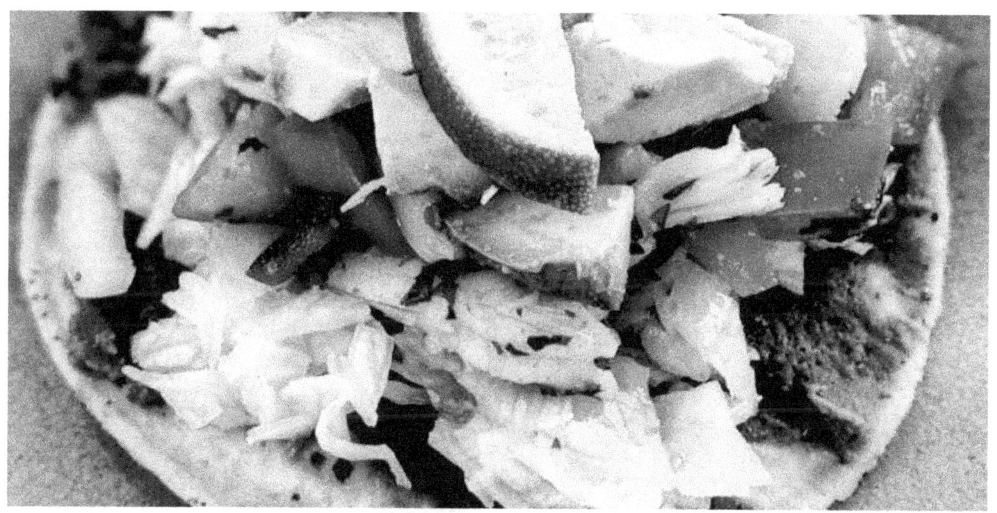

INGREDIENTS

1 lb. cooked shrimp (You could even use frozen, thawed shrimp.)

1 cup roma tomatoes, deseeded and diced (1/2-inch pieces)

3 jalapeños, seeded and finely chopped

1 small red onion diced (1/2-inch pieces)

1 can black refried beans

3 tbsp fresh cilantro finely chopped, juice of 3 limes, juice of 2 lemons, 1 tbsp white vinegar, 1 tbsp hot sauce, 2 tsp garlic salt, 1 avocado, 6 tostadas

DIRECTIONS

1. Chop the shrimp into large pieces and set aside.
2. In a glass bowl, combine tomatoes, jalapeños, red onion, and cilantro. Add in chopped shrimp. Add in lemon juice, lime juice, white vinegar, hot sauce, and garlic salt. Toss a few times with a large spoon until everything is well combined. Refrigerate for 30 minutes, stirring occasionally.
3. After the ceviche has been refrigerated, add in the avocado.
4. Assemble the tostadas: Top each tostada with a spoonful of black refried beans, shredded lettuce and the ceviche mixture. Serve immediately. BOOM!

Recipe inspired by: www.mariahspleasingplates.com

BERRY CHOCOLATE *Oats*

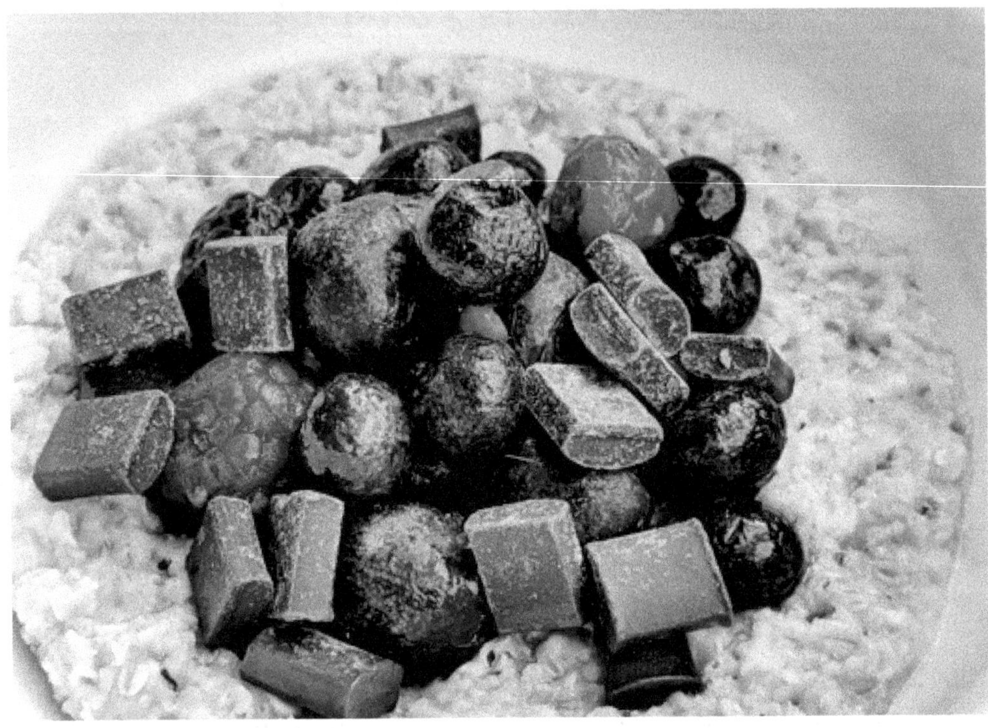

INGREDIENTS

1/3 cup oats

1/3 cup flaxmilk + protein (or whatever you have)

3/4 tbsp chocolate chips

5-8 grams Agave

Splash Vanilla or Almond extract (I used almond)

1/4 cup mixed berries (or your fruit of choice)

DIRECTIONS

1. Combine all ingredients in a mug, stir and store overnight.
2. Heat SLOWLY (30 seconds at a time) and mix in between heating, you may also need to add some extra water or milk depending on how thick you like your oats!

I am ALWAYS trying new variations of overnight oats, and this one takes the cake!

Huevos Rancheros

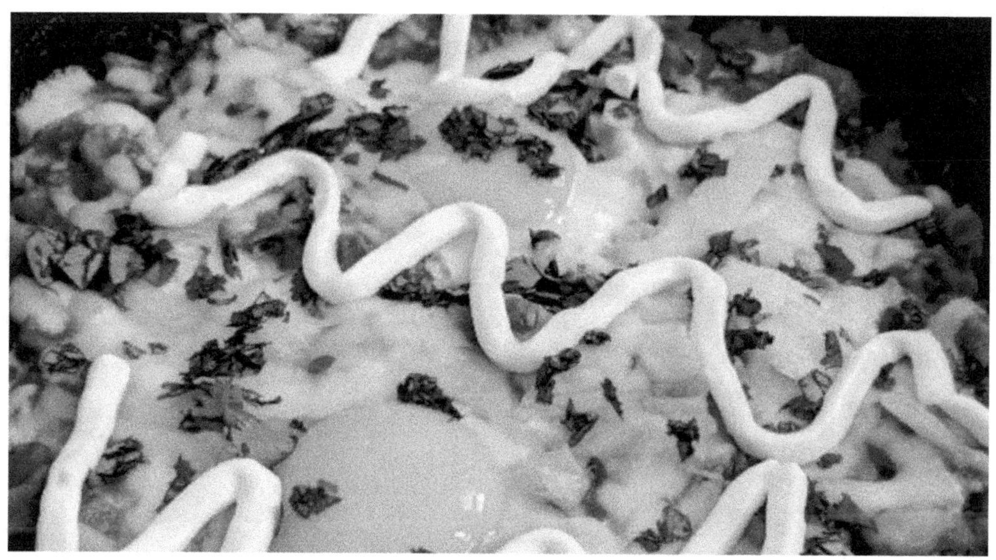

INGREDIENTS

1 egg

1/2 cup Rotel

Garlic

2 tbsp fat-free Fage

1/4 cup red or orange pepper

1/4 cup onion

1/3 cup fat-free refried beans

Optional toppings:
lettuce and/or cilantro

DIRECTIONS

1. Spray skillet with cooking spray and heat to medium.
2. Add onions and peppers and sauté until soft. Add in however much garlic you like. Sauté for a minute or so.
3. Add the refried beans and the Rotel and cook for a few minutes.
4. Make a well in the beans mixture and add the egg, then cook until your liking.
5. Leave in skillet for serving and top with cilantro, lettuce, fat-free Fage and enjoy!

MACROS PER SERVING: 23C/5F/18P

PROTEIN *Waffle*

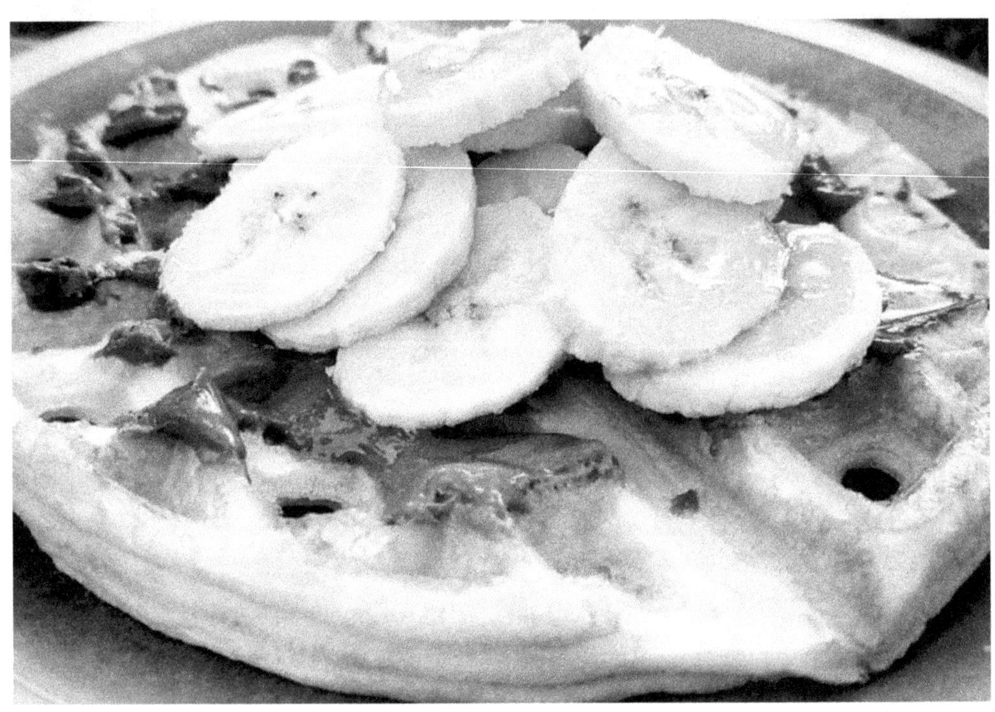

INGREDIENTS

1 scoop Protein powder (I always use Vanilla)

20 grams egg whites

1 tsp baking powder

3 tbsp water or milk

DIRECTIONS

1. Add all ingredients and mix well.
2. Heat waffle iron and spray with cooking spray.
3. Pour batter into waffle iron.
4. Serve with spray butter or PB2, and sugar free syrup or agave!

THE ULTIMATE *Hash*

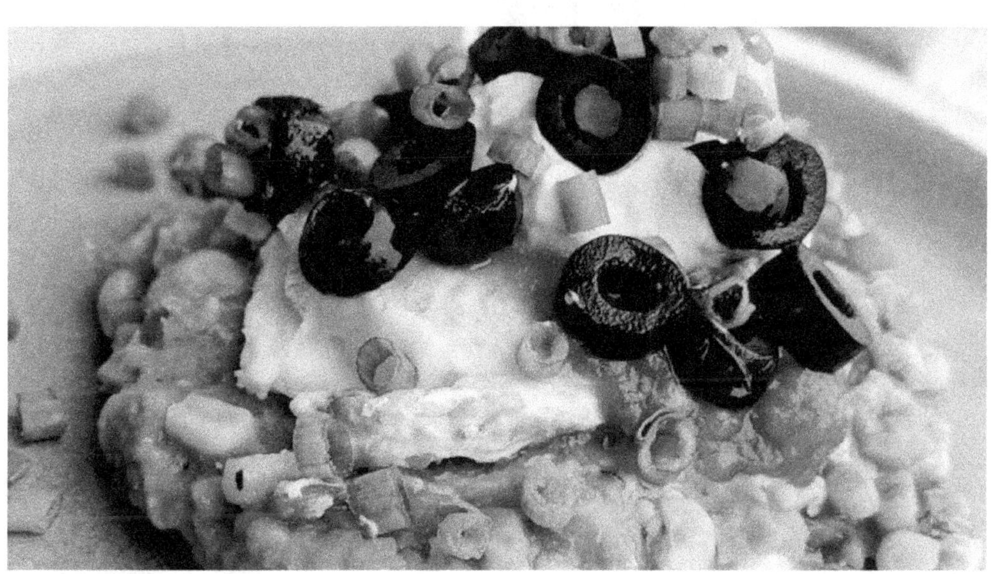

INGREDIENTS

1/4 cup Fat free or low-fat refried beans

1 egg

2 tbsp light sour cream

1 tbsp black olives

Salsa

Scallions

2 tbps Trader Joe's corn salsa

DIRECTIONS

1. Heat beans and corn salsa in skillet.
2. Make a well in the center. After a few minutes, crack the egg in the well and cook.
3. Move to a plate and top with toppings!

THROW TOGETHER
Breakfast Tacos

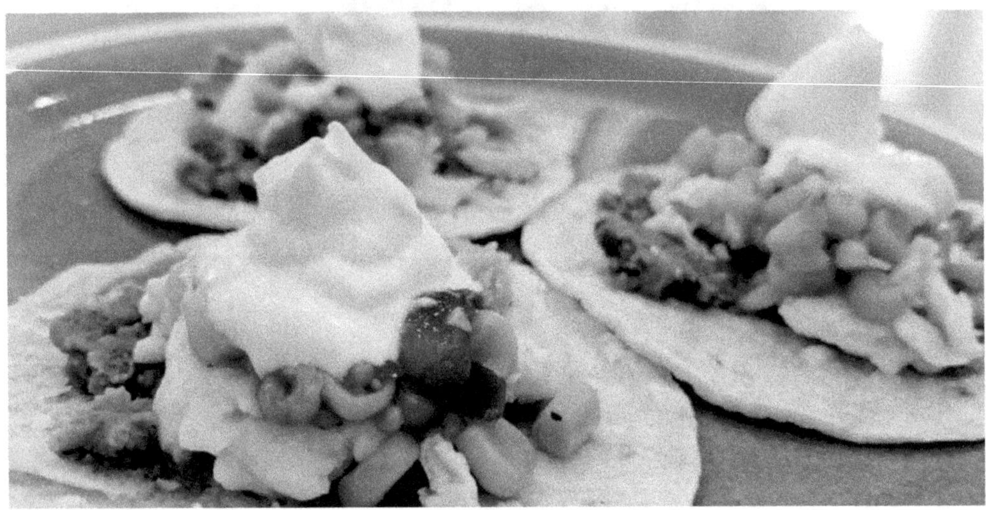

INGREDIENTS

1/4 cup Refried black beans

2 street taco sized corn tortillas

1 egg

2 tbsp light sour cream

2 tbsp Trader Joe's corn salsa

DIRECTIONS

1. Cook egg however you like.
2. Warm up tortillas in a wet paper towel in the microwave for 20 seconds.
3. Spread bean mixture on tortillas, add egg and corn salsa, and heat for 15-20 more seconds.
4. Top with sour cream and devour.

You could even add some Crock-Pot chicken if you have it prepped, to up the protein!

TASTY TUNA
Pasta Salad

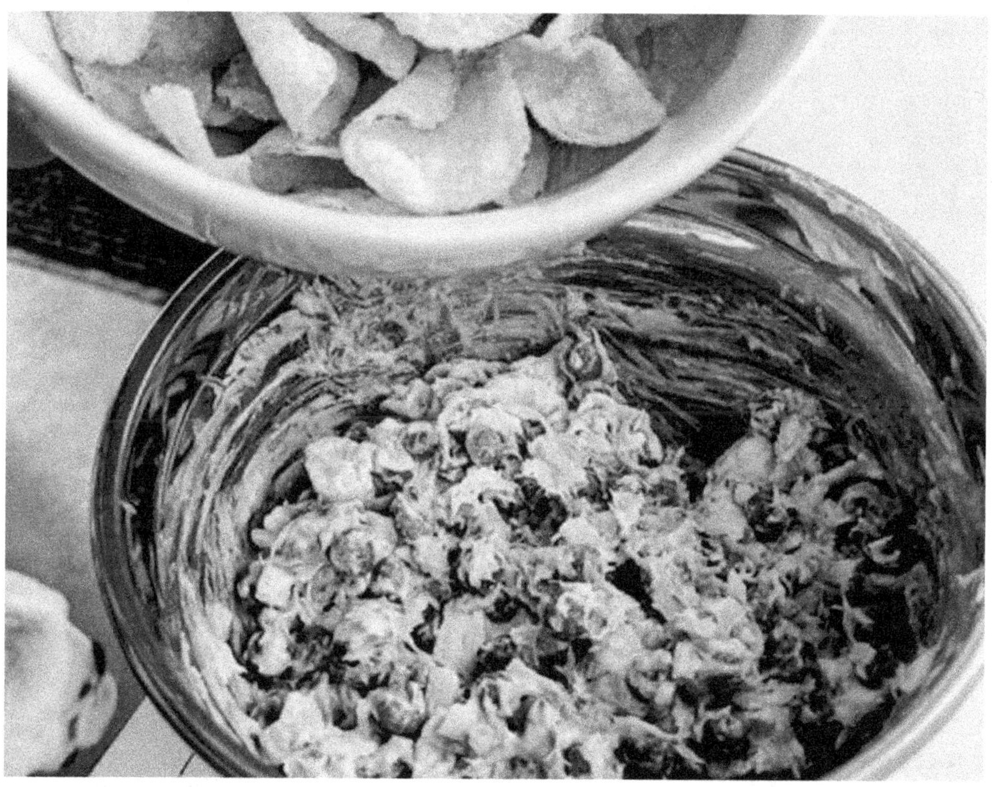

INGREDIENTS

1 packet Bumblebee tuna (I like the lemon pepper flavor.)

1/2 cup frozen peas

1 oz fat-free Fage yogurt

1/2 tbsp honey mustard

1/2 oz cheddar cheese

1/8 cup pasta

DIRECTIONS

1. Combine all ingredients.
2. Serve with 1/2 oz sea salt and vinegar kettle chips for dipping---BOOM!

Recipe inspired by: Grace Ramos

MACROS PER SERVING: 35C/13F/30P

PUMPKIN PROTEIN *Muffins*

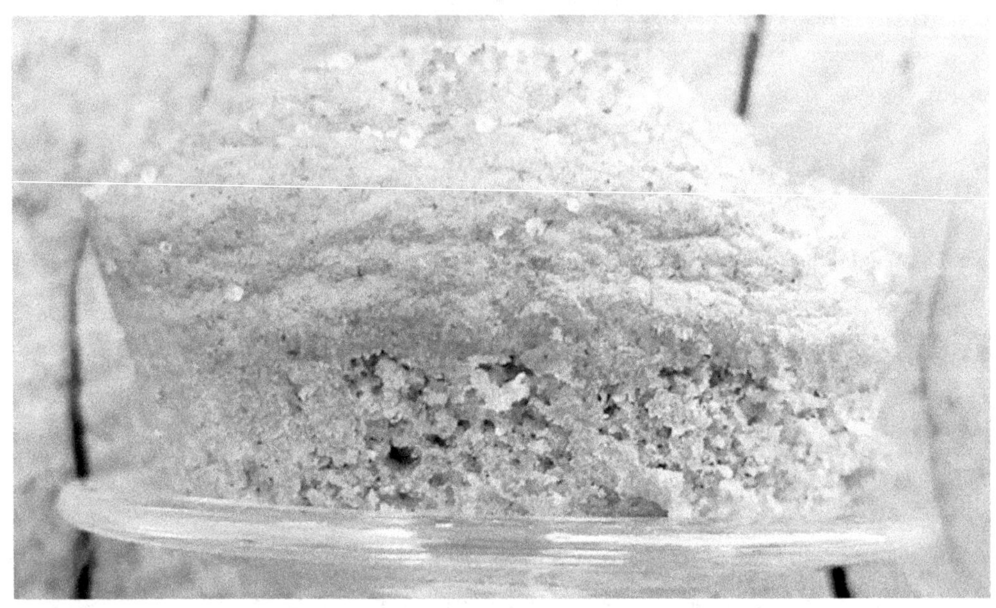

INGREDIENTS

1 ¾ cup GF oats

1 tsp baking soda, 2 tsp baking powder, ¼ tsp salt, 1 ½ tsp cinnamon, ½ tsp pumpkin pie spice, ½ cup swerve (or sugar baking substitute)

¼ cup vanilla flavored protein powder (heaping scoop)

1 cup canned pumpkin

½ cup unsweetened applesauce

½ cup fat-free Fage

6 tbsp liquid egg whites

Optional add-ins for family: chocolate chips, pecans, almonds, walnuts, raisins

DIRECTIONS

1. Preheat oven to 350. Line 12 muffin tins with liners or spray with nonstick spray.

3. Blend oats until smooth, then add other dry ingredients. Add all other ingredients to mixer and blend well, except for add-ins.

4. Divide mixture among muffin tins, place in oven.

5. Bake for 15-20 minutes, or until tops are lightly golden brown.

   *Batter is super moist; toothpick may not come out clean.

6. Cool muffins before removing from pan.

Recipe from: www.kimscravings.com

MACROS PER MUFFIN: 18C/1F/6P

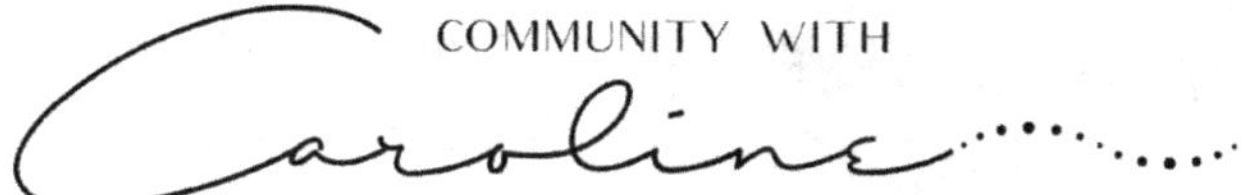

COMMUNITY TESTIMONIALS

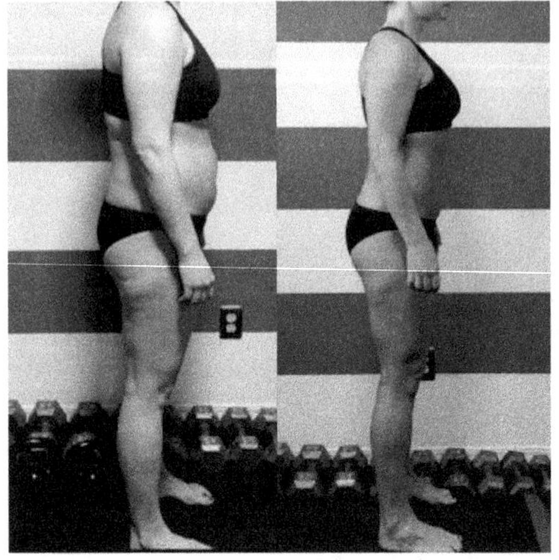

I've been following you and watching you, and I see the realness in you that I haven't seen in the millions of other fitness accounts. Thank you for these live videos that share the realness and say the tough things that we all need to hear, to motivate us in the right ways and keep us on track. You are doing a great thing and I am so glad I found you!"

Nellie Y.

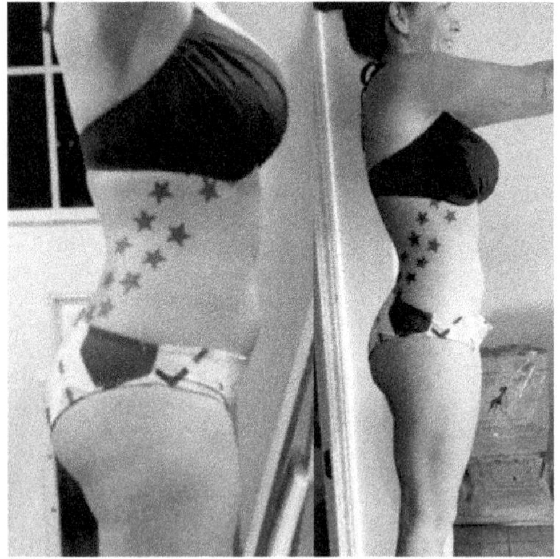

A year ago today I was so defeated. I just want you to know that you are doing amazing things for people. Confidence and happiness are not things that you can put a price tag on or even explain, but you are giving so many women both of those things! From the bottom of my heart, thank you!"

Ashley S.

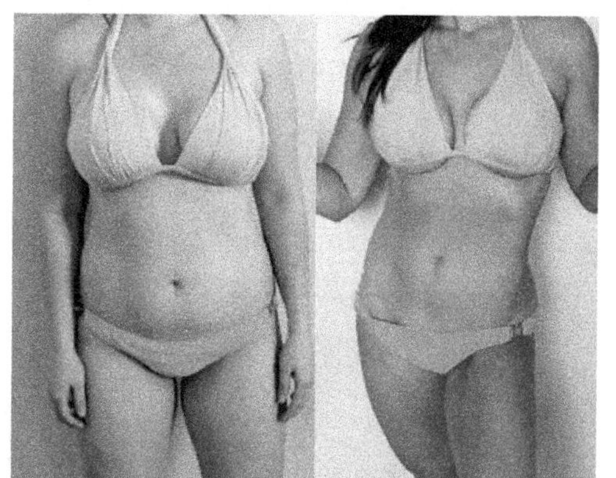

“

I really don't have the words to say except ‘THANK YOU!’ Never in a million years did I think I would lose that weight. I always just accepted that this would be my size forever, boy was I wrong! I had no idea about what was in food before and all it took was learning to read food labels and exercise portion control! This process has been a lot easier than I thought, THANK YOU!”

Kelsey C.

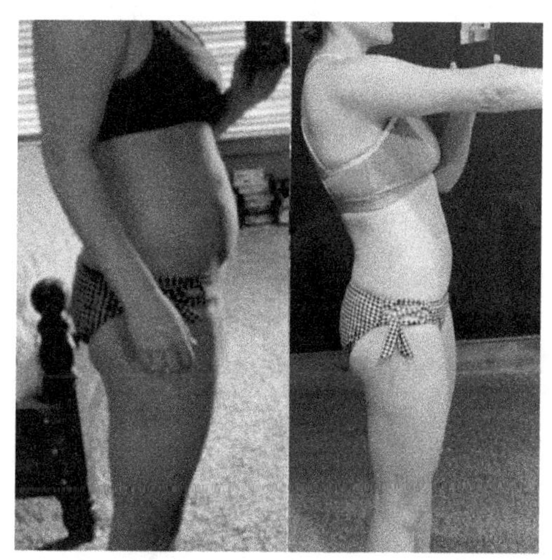

“

I went backpacking in Yellowstone and enjoyed every minute of it! I didn't go hiking with my husband last year because I knew I'd be miserable and feel disgusted with myself the whole time. This year I was able to go and LOVED IT! I just wanted to say ‘thank you’ AGAIN for helping me to get where I am. I still know I have a ways to go, but my love for life right now exceeds 1000 times what it did last year at this time. THANK YOU!”

Natalie H.

Battled an
Auto-Immune
Disease
July 2016
Feb 2019
Jul 2014

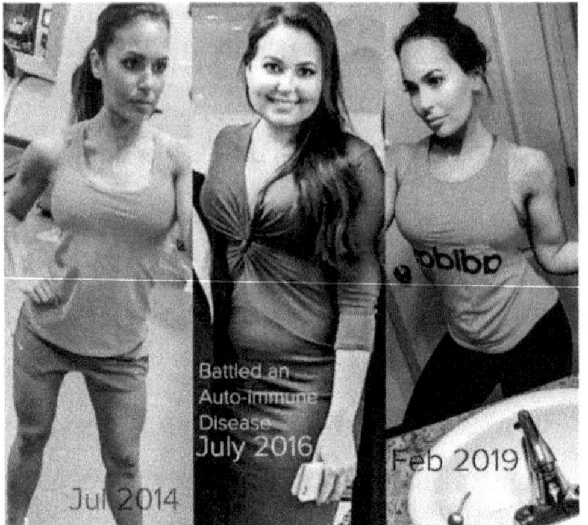

"This is the first time in a LONG time that I have seen this kind of definition in my arms/upper body. It is also the first time that I'm not feeling completely depleted of energy or the will to continue after 12 weeks. It is the first time I've worked with someone who created a flexible meal plan for me (I literally look forward to each meal). She is equally invested in my mental progress in relation to my self-image as she is my physical progress. Caroline is the REAL DEAL!"

Jackie V.

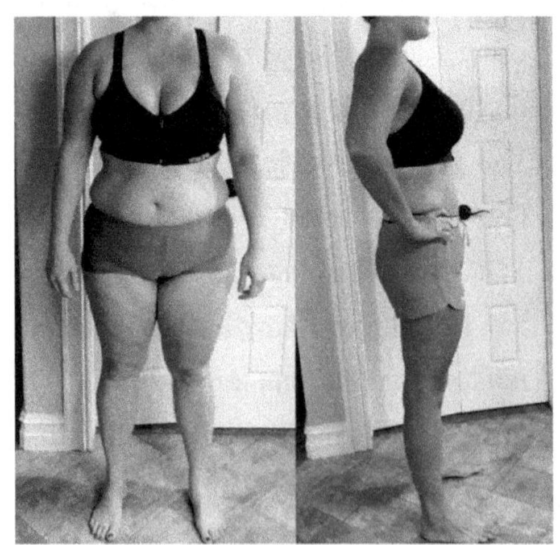

"You have lit the fire inside of me and given me the tools to succeed and nothing is going to stop me now! I know I will hit speed bumps but now I know that it's just a bump and not a wall."

Ammie J.

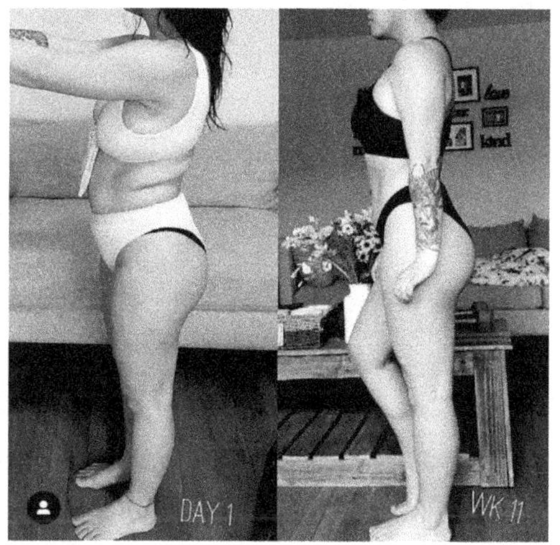

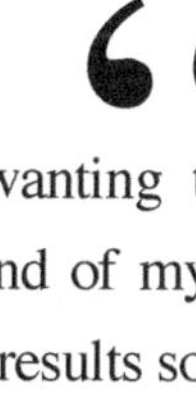

I wasn't wanting to share my results until the end of my program, but I am loving my results so far so I had to share them! Big thanks to my coach, Caroline Mathias for helping me get started on my diet. She is amazing! And when I say 'amazing' I literally mean 'AMAZING!' I've gained 40 lbs in the last 3 years and I was not comfortable in bathing suits or tight clothing. I was miserable and I had to stop feeling this way. I then found Caroline on Facebook through a mutual friend. She is very specific and will help you get through the cravings, really everything. She is GREAT!"

Nanncy Y.

CPSIA information can be obtained
at www.ICGtesting.com
Printed in the USA
BVHW041003010320
573478BV00008B/96

9 780578 630069